# Christ-Centered Holistic Health:
## Achieving Optimal Wellness through Balance

Charlotte Eliopoulos

This book is dedicated to my husband George Considine
for his support and encouragement.

# CONTENTS

# CHAPTER 1
# INTRODUCTION

**My Personal Journey To Holistic Health**

Like many authors, my journey to the final destination of this book involved travel through some familiar paths, the discovery of new avenues, bumpy detours, and surprising intersections.  I have been a health care professional for decades, beginning my career as a nurse.  By professional standards I'm considered successful:  I've written several textbooks, lectured and consulted internationally, gained respect as a leader in my specialty of gerontological nursing, and been able to hold my own in medical circles.

A major life-changing twist in my journey occurred in the 1990s.  At that time, I was feeling quite competent and confident, on top of my game. Angelo, the man to whom I was married at the time, and I were riding high, enjoying a satisfying, happy life.  With children grown and some investment income to support us, Angelo had opted for an early retirement to pursue his passion for art.  We traveled, collected art and antiques, and enjoyed an active social life.

 In the midst of what seemed to be an ideal life, Angelo developed some vague back pain.  At first he wrote it off to a muscle strain, but as it continued to worsen, he finally conceded to my request that he seek medical attention.  A CAT scan revealed the unexpected:  Angelo had a tumor in his liver.  A biopsy confirmed that it was not only a malignancy, but a rare form of cancer that had no effective treatment options.  Couched in sophisticated medical jargon---much the same that I had tossed to patients over the years--- the message was conveyed that although some chemotherapy could be tried, my 54 year-old husband most likely would not see his 55th birthday.

At the time of Angelo's diagnosis I was a seeker.  I sensed there was a "higher being" but wasn't quite sure what that meant.  My independent attempts at reading the Bible left me empty.  I had not known any Christians in an intimate way; the only persons who I associated with Christianity were those who attended church on Sunday but then lived sinful lives the rest of the time.  To complicate matters, Angelo was a professed atheist who had little patience with my interest in exploring God's presence in my life.  So here we were, facing a major crisis in the absence of a relationship with the Lord.

From a clinical perspective, Angelo received state-of-the-art care.  Chemotherapy was efficiently instilled, laboratory tests closely monitored, and scans properly interpreted.  All the textbook standards were met.  Yet, none of these expert practitioners seemed to notice the profoundly depressed, spiritually distressed man who was before them.  Angelo could not make sense of this tragedy.  He viewed each day as a cruel reminder that he was being robbed of the life he had so enjoyed.  Without a belief in a hereafter, the here and now was unbearable.

A ray of light did shine into Angelo's life in the person of a gentle man named John.  John, who belonged to a church that my sister-in-law attended, had a ministry of visiting the sick.  When my sister-in-law phoned and suggested that John visit Angelo in the hospital, I was enthusiastic but thought there was a 50-50 chance that Angelo would throw him out of the room.  Most likely out of respect for my sister-in-law, Angelo agreed to John's visit.

The visit went surprisingly well.  Angelo and John were both of Greek descent and chatted about several mutual interests.  No mention of God was made until John was ready to leave.  "Can I pray for you before I go?" John directly inquired.  I held my breath, anticipating that Angelo would have a few choice words for John.  I could barely believe my ears when I heard the response, "Well, okay, but don't expect me to be saying or doing anything while you do that."  With that, John offered a simple, sweet prayer and left.

As the months passed, John maintained contact with Angelo.  He would phone, chat, and witness to Angelo.  I doubted that this was having any impact on Angelo's spiritual life, but was appreciative for the opportunity for Angelo to enjoy the relationship.

Meanwhile, the struggle between being the health care professional and devastated wife watching her husband dying was tremendous for me.  Because of my nursing background, the physicians were quite open with me ---painfully so.  They often pulled me on the side, reviewing dismal test results or discussing the latest organ invaded by the relentless cancer cells.  Ripped apart inside, I plastered a smile on my face and exchanged clinical opinions as though we were talking about a malfunctioning car rather than my husband's dwindling life.   I asked little of friends and family---after all, I *was* a nurse and accustomed to handling these things.  In addition to the toll that 24-hour caregiving was taking on my physical health, I was emotionally drained and spiritually pained.  It was at this time that I began to feel the stirrings of a spiritual awakening.  I began to speak with God on a regular basis and search the Bible for direction.  And I knew, very definitely, that I was being sustained on a power that exceeded my own capabilities---a power I believed to be God.

Angelo's condition declined to the point that I knew death was imminent.  Although there continued to be no talk of faith from Angelo, I felt it was important that he not die without having a least one special prayer, so I phoned and asked John, the closest thing to a man of the cloth I knew, to visit.  John graciously agreed to come the next day. I told him to phone before he came so that I would provide directions, as he had never visited Angelo at our home.

The morning of John's scheduled visit Angelo fell into a coma.  Despite my turning him, injecting him, and trying to arouse him, he was unresponsive.  I phoned John and advised him not to bother to come.

As evening came Angelo's brothers and I sat in the family room that housed Angelo's hospital bed, waiting, hoping  for some last opportunity to communicate with him.  Except for his slow, rattling breaths, he offered little sign of life.

Our quiet vigil was interrupted by a knock on the door.  I was surprised to have a visitor on this cold, rainy December evening and even more surprised when I opened the door to see John standing there.  As I mentioned, he had never visited our home and it was not the easiest location to find.  In reaction to the stunned look on my face John offered, "I wanted to see Angelo."

"Sure," I responded, "you can visit.  But, understand that he is not responding."

With a calm assurance John entered the family room and Angelo's brothers and I exited to the adjacent room to provide some privacy for the visit.  As I was leaving the room I heard Angelo 's voice say "John, is that you?"  I was startled, as these were the first words he had uttered all day.

As my brothers-in-law and I observed from the next room we saw Angelo raise his arms and interact with John, although we weren't able to hear what was spoken.  About ten minutes later, John walked to us and calmly said, "He is alright now."  Before I could get my wits together to inquire about what transpired, John was gone.  Immediately my brothers-in-law and I went to Angelo, only to find him again unresponsive.  To say we were baffled would be an understatement.

That night Angelo died.  It wasn't until months later that I learned that Angelo accepted Christ during that last visit with John.

Later, John shared that he was relieved when I phoned to cancel the visit.  He was tired from a hard day of work and relaxing in the warmth of his home seemed much more appealing than venturing out in the harsh weather.  "But, I just couldn't rest," shared John.  "The Holy Spirit was stirring me until I knew that I couldn't find peace until I visited Angelo.  I didn't understand why at the time, just that I needed to be with him."  Fortunately, John heeded the direction he was given.

The example of the way the Lord worked through John and my need to make sense of my scrambled life helped to fuel my spiritual growth.  I still wasn't sure what it meant, but I did sense a need for a connection with something, someone greater than myself.  Further, I was devastated by the lack of spiritual care offered to Angelo.  My honest self-evaluation caused me to see that I was just as guilty as Angelo's caregivers in ignoring the spiritual aspects of health and healing; I became committed to change the course of my career to support a model of care that respected the importance and interrelationship of mind, body, and spirit.

I found the journey into holistic care to be an exciting one---certainly more colorful and varied than the roads I traveled in mainstream medicine.  The practices and practitioners addressed the whole person---body, mind, and spirit.  Healing, rather than curing was emphasized.  Instead of passively looking to health care professionals to direct and treat them, individuals assumed an active role in their health and healing.  Multicultural healing therapies were honored.  And very importantly, there was acknowledgement that one's spiritual well-being was as important to health as diet and exercise.

In the midst of my travels into holism, I became a Christian.  As I said, I knew something was stirring within and my holistic practitioner colleagues generously sprinkled their conversations with talk of *spirit* which further stimulated my appetite.  However, it wasn't until I became friends with a neighbor who happened to be a Christian that I began to understand the significance of a relationship with Jesus.  My neighbor George and I had a casual friendship until an evening when we shared dinner and realized that we had enough in common to date.  In a short time we both knew that feelings beyond a neighborly friendship were brewing.  It was then that George sat me down and dropped a bombshell on me:  "You've got to know that I am a born-again Christian," he said,  "and that my relationship with Jesus Christ always will  come first."  Quite honestly, I didn't know what to make of this.

Until that time my image of born-again Christians was less than flattering.  I viewed them as narrow-minded, dull people who existed in a limited world.  Yet, here was my friend George--- seemingly normal, intelligent, and fun---ascribing this label to himself.  My curiosity was piqued.  God was very kind in blessing me with an open mind and heart to learn more about this "relationship with Jesus Christ" business.

As time progressed, George introduced me to his church, Grace Fellowship, an evangelical nondenominational one in Timonium Maryland.  Here I met dynamic, bright, spirited people who had a passion for the Lord.  It was as though a veil had been lifted from my eyes as I began to see clearly the impact that a relationship with Christ could have in one's life.  Soon thereafter, I accepted Jesus Christ into my life.  Bible studies, fellowship with other Christians, and a call to ministry helped to deepen my walk with Christ---and still do.

George and I eventually married.  Although I considered myself happily married to Angelo, my marriage to George has a richness that was absent in my previous marriage in that Jesus Christ is at the core of our relationship.

In the midst of my accepting and developing a relationship with Christ, I also was traveling further down the path of holistic health in my professional life.  Angelo's illness vividly showed me that health and healing entailed more than concern for the physical body.  I began to explore the literature on holistic health, attended whatever seminars I could, and committed to becoming a holistic practitioner---i.e., one who addresses the body, mind, and spirit of a person as indivisible components of a complex whole.  I obtained a PhD in natural health and doctor of naturopathy degrees and used this knowledge to assist individuals with chronic health conditions or those interested in improving health.  Now I find I am as interested in their spiritual well-being (e.g., their relationship with God, avenues for receiving and offering love, sources of purpose, meaning, and hope) as I am in their mental and physical status.  My intent is that they will prevent problems from developing and identify the factors that contribute to their disorders rather than just treat symptoms once they arise.  The "interventions" I use to supplement conventional health practices are likely to include prayer, listening, facilitating the patching of relationships, offering a massage, recommending an herb, supporting, and teaching.  Often, I partner with people to help them explore the purpose of their illness and suffering.  Basically, I tend to their bodies, minds, and spirits.

## The Meaning of Holistic Health

Holistic health refers to the integration of the mind, body, and spirit to create a dynamic whole that is more powerful and significant than the sum of the parts. In other words, 1+1+1= 5 or 10 or more. A holistic view recognizes that the various aspects of an individual---physical, mental, and spiritual---profoundly affected each other, being interwoven and indivisible.

Although the term holistic health gained popularity in the last quarter of the 20th Century, God revealed the relationship of body, mind, and spirit from the earliest of times. Solomon declared that *a cheerful heart is good medicine but a crushed spirit dries up the bones* (Proverbs 17:22) acknowledging that our mood impacts our physical body. Jesus Christ interacted with people holistically. One example in which this was shown is the story of the woman who had suffered with hemorrhaging for twelve years and was healed by touching Jesus' garments (Mark 5:25-34). Jesus told her that her faith had made her well, offering the message that our spiritual state in being faithful to him was of utmost importance and could affect our physical condition. Jesus was intent on healing the spirit and not just concerned about physical or mental symptoms.

Scripture is filled with wisdom pertaining to health. Rather than possessing the perfect body or being free from illness or disability, Biblically-based health implies:

- Being committed and obedient to God
- Honoring the temple with which God has blessed us
- Accepting illness as having purpose in God's plan

By dying for our sins Jesus opened the road to eternal life for us. What will be the condition of the body, mind, and spirit that we offer Him? Will we have been good stewards of these precious gifts?

## Observations About Holistic Health and Christianity

The professional associations in which I have become involved include those with an integrative care and holistic focus. In fact, I became active in and president of the American Holistic Nurses' Association which immersed me in the holistic arena quite heavily. Within these circles there is much emphasis on the significance of *spirit* in one's life. However, the source of spirit encountered tends to be open game. Upon exploring popular literature on wellness and holistic health, you could get the impression that the secrets to an optimum life can be found through clearing energy fields, meditating with a maharishi, balancing chakras, chanting mantras, and getting in touch with a past life. Much of the holistic health movement has been influenced heavily by Eastern, Native American, and New Age philosophies. Channeling universal life energies from unknown origins, utilizing spirits of the dead, and placing one's faith in an object or practitioner are among the practices often associated with holistic health.

Although colorful and interesting, the practices associated with popular holistic health philosophies present challenges for Christians because they are dishonoring to God. As a result, many Christians have determined that *holistic health* is incompatible with their faith and steered away from anything associated with the term. Christian acquaintances, when learning of my professional background, have challenged me about my involvement in this arena.  Some have adamantly stated that they would have nothing to do with anything labeled "holistic".  In workshops that I've presented to Christian audiences, there have been a few participants who left during discussions of meditation and herbal therapies.   Some church members have asked to meet with me privately and confided their use of alternative therapies, fearful that they were committing a sin by using these modalities.   While some holistic health practices can be dishonoring to the Lord, particularly those that call on universal energy sources as means of healing, there are holistic health principles and practices that are not only consistent with Scripture, but quite honoring to God. Unfortunately, confusion, fear, and lack of knowledge concerning God-honoring health practices have resulted in some Christians being inattentive to practices that could enhance their health, glorify God, and enable them to be more effective servants of the Lord.

Another consequence of Christians' steering clear of holistic health circles is that Jesus Christ has had a weak presence, if any at all, when spirituality has been discussed in this arena, thereby depriving many people from learning about a relationship that can change the course of their lives.  My experience and friendships with holistic health practitioners have convinced me that they are not insensitive people who have made a well-researched decision to reject Christianity; rather, they have not been afforded the opportunity to learn about a relationship with Jesus Christ.  Many have had unpleasant experiences with organized religion and equate that to Christianity.  Others have never had anyone share the Good News with them.  (Being a person who lived forty plus years before anyone witnessed to me, I can appreciate the ignorance about Christianity that one can have.)  For the most part, these are spiritually hungry people seeking a path of meaning. Unfortunately, the buffet that they are offered from the best-selling literature and charismatic leaders of the holistic movement provides generous portions of spirituality that often doesn't even include Jesus Christ as an after dinner mint.  Rather than retreat from holistic health circles with fear and disdain, Christians may better serve and glorify God by shining a light within these groups that clearly shows the optimum model for holistic health is *Christ-centered.*

This book offers suggestions for achieving holistic health from a Christian perspective.  Rather than following the latest diet craze or firming abs at the gym, health will be considered as an abundant way of life centered in Christ.  Using the acronym **BALANCE**, the book will aid you in improving your health by:
> **B**elieving you can achieve an abundant, empowered life so that you can strengthen positive lifestyle habits and change those patterns that prevent you from achieving optimum health
> **A**ssessing the current state of your body, mind, and spirit so that you'll understand your unique capabilities and deficits
> **L**earning about the meaning of good health and habits that foster it
> **A**cquiring positive habits that are tailored to your unique body, mind, spirit and lifestyle
> **N**urturing yourself so that you enhance the ability of your mind and spirit to promote good health
> **C**onnecting in a better way with yourself, significant others in your life, and Jesus Christ
> **E**xperiencing and learning to appreciate life's blessings so that you can live abundantly

You will be guided in reflecting on your personal habits and developing individualized plans that you can incorporate into your life to improve your health.  This will require some honest self-evaluation and work on your part---nothing worthwhile comes easily.  However, the results can be exciting and life changing.

# CHAPTER 2
# BELIEVE YOU CAN ACHIEVE
# A HEALTHY AND ABUNDANT LIFE

*What does it mean to you to believe in something?*

Usually you have faith or confidence in something in which you believe. You trust that it can be depended upon to be true and often proceed with actions confidently based on that understanding. For example, you believed that the chair you are sitting on could hold your weight and seated yourself without hesitancy. You acted based on your beliefs.

Your values provide a frame of reference for your beliefs. Values consist of your standards and that which has worth to you. They offer meaning and direction. The Bible provides the foundation for the values Christians hold.

The state of your health can be influenced significantly by the beliefs you hold and, in turn, your health-related beliefs can be influenced significantly by the worldview of the society in which you live. You may have given the relationship between the worldview and your beliefs little thought, but it has impacted you. When it comes to matters of health, our society has valued the scientific approach---the *biomedical model*---characterized by the following:

- *Mechanism:* the human body is explained in terms of physics and chemistry and considered to operate much like a machine. Health is determined by physical structure and function, and disease is a malfunction of the physical part. Malfunctions and malformations are undesirable. Disease is treated by repairing the malformed or malfunctioning organ or system with physical or chemical interventions (e.g., drugs, surgery). God has no role in one's health state or healing, and dysfunction and deformity serve no purpose.

- *Materialism:* the human body and its state of health are influenced only by what can be seen and measured. Illness is caused by a physical malfunction and is addressed by concrete treatments. One's emotional and spiritual states have no impact on health and healing.

- *Reductionism*: the human body is viewed in terms of isolated parts.  Treatment of a health condition addresses the individual organ or system rather than the whole being.  One can have good health by having body systems that function well, despite spiritual state.

Within these belief systems, you could be considered healthy in the absence of a relationship with God.  Further, illness, deformity, and disability serve no purpose.

In recent years the biomedical model has been challenged by a *holistic model* which is based on the beliefs that:

- Each person is a highly individualized being made of body, mind, and spirit.
- A person's body, mind, and spirit are interrelated.
- Health is judged not merely by the absence of disease, but by wholeness and harmony of the body, mind, and spirit.
- The treatment of disease addresses and utilizes the resources of the body, mind, and spirit.
- Disease can serve a purpose.

As you probably can see, this model appears more consistent with Christian values.  Discernment is necessary, however, as in some holistic health circles Jesus Christ is not considered the supreme being guiding one's spirit and spiritual care could consist of interventions inconsistent with Christian beliefs (this will be discussed later).  For a Christian, a balanced, healthy life is a choice based upon the beliefs that God:

- wants the best for you
  *I am the Lord your God, who brought you out of Egypt so that you would no longer be slaves to the Egyptians; I broke the bars of your yoke and enabled you to walk with heads held high.*  Leviticus 26:13
- provides you with that which you need
  *The Lord will guide you always; He will satisfy your needs in a sun-scorched land and will strengthen your frame.*  Isaiah 58:11
- strengthens you through the indwelling of the Holy Spirit
  *I can do everything through Him who gives me strength.*  Philippians 4:13
- desires you to honor the life he has given you by taking care of it
  *Do you not know that your body is a temple of the Holy Spirit, who is in you, whom you have received from God?*  1 Corinthians 6:19
- has plans for you that you may not fully understand at present
  *"For I know the plans I have for you," declares the Lord…* Jeremiah 29:11

If you're like many people, at some time in your life you've made impressive plans for self-improvement on New Year's Eve, only to have them abandoned by mid-February.  Many intentions to improve health are doomed from the start because of the lack of belief in the ability to change or succeed.  This lack of belief is couched in comments like *"I can't find time in my schedule to shop for groceries, much less build in an exercise program or relaxation exercises,"* or, *"My mother was overweight and her mother before her, so I guess I just inherited their genes."*  Excuses, blame, and rationalizations often prevent us from taking positive actions and altering the landscape of our health.  Sometimes we stay in unhealthy patterns because we believe them to offer more comfort and security than the alternatives, much like the resistance of the oppressed people  Moses led through the desert who were tempted to remain in the security of slavery rather than risk a hard journey to the Promised Land.

**Self-Evaluation**

Prior to launching your effort to improve your health, it is helpful to examine the beliefs that influence your health behaviors.  The following questions will guide you in this self-evaluation.

1. What does *good health* mean to you?
2. To what degree do you see your health state as a matter of fate?
3. To what degree are you willing to change each of the following to improve your health:
   - Eating habits?
   - Amount of activity and exercise?
   - Leisure activities?
   - Quality of relationships?
   - Lifestyle?
   - Allocation of time for prayer and solitude?
4. Deep down, do you think that you won't be affected by eating poorly, failing to exercise, shortchanging your sleep requirements, and skipping personal quiet time?
5. In regard to diet, activities, and relationships, did your family promote behaviors that ran contrary to good health practices (e.g., eating high-fat foods, tolerating abusive relationships, ignoring drunkenness of a family member)?
6. Do the benefits of looking and feeling better outweigh the sacrifices you may need to make in forfeiting unhealthy practices?
7. Do you think it is selfish to spend time relaxing and exercising, or  to refuse to engage in social functions with friends and family who are draining?
8. Do you believe you can influence your current state of health?

**Meaning of Health**

For years, health was assumed to mean the absence of disease, but that definition has fallen by the wayside.  You may realize from experiences in your own life that you can be free from any formal diagnosis of a health condition, yet not be feeling or functioning at your best.  Now, as mentioned, health is viewed in terms of harmony and vitality of the body, mind, and spirit.  This broader description implies that when you are healthy you:

   - awaken each day with enthusiasm, energy, a sense of purpose, and a will to live
   - connect with people and nature
   - love and allow yourself to be loved
   - accept and offer forgiveness
   - have a relationship with the Lord.

With this perspective, you can be healthy despite having a disease or disability.  This was displayed to me many years ago when I was a teenage "Candy-Striper" in the long-term care section of what was then Baltimore City Hospital.  This was the city's "charity hospital" that cared for people too poor to seek care elsewhere during these pre-Medicaid days.  On one of the dingy, large wards lived a man named Charlie Toye.  Mr. Toye had resided on the ward for many years before I met him and had no family.  Further, he was quadriplegic and totally dependent on others for the most basic of needs.  I had never seen a person like this before, and my teenage mind pondered how anyone could bear this condition.  But as the weeks passed, I noticed that Mr. Toye's room seemed to be a magnet for staff.  Housekeepers, nursing assistants, nurses, and maintenance workers would approach his bedside looking tired and beaten, but depart with new energy and smiles.  Although he couldn't lift a finger, Mr. Toye could touch others through his attentive listening, kind words, and warm heart.  This motionless man who couldn't raise food to his own mouth fed the souls of those he encountered.  And he must have gotten back what he gave as he was consistently cheerful, optimistic, and positive.  Years later, after completing nursing school, I returned to this hospital to work and found Mr. Toye still holding court with employees, still lifting spirits, still displaying joy.  I believe Mr. Toye enjoyed a high level of holistic health.

**Responsibility for Health**

Viewing health as a matter of fate causes you to feel powerless in your ability to change the course of your life.  *"It's out of my hands," "I never have any luck."* and *"You can't change the cards you've been dealt"* are comments reflecting a fatalistic view of health.  Granted, there are some realities that you cannot change, such as being born with a developmental disability, and God does have a plan for you that may involve living with certain conditions.  But, you can exercise tremendous power to maximize your God-given potential by taking care of your body, mind, and spirit.  Placing responsibility for your health on fate makes no more sense than trusting the oil change in your car to fate, rather than conscious effort.  God has given you life, health, and resources, and expects you to use them wisely.

You may understand what good health practices are and have a desire to improve your health, but be unwilling to make sacrifices.  *"I'll gain weight if I stop smoking." "If I no longer stop for a drink after work I'll lose contact with my friends." "I've got several small kids; I don't have time to indulge in an aerobics class."* Although you have the potential to change and adopt healthy practices, you must have the desire to do so.

Consistently following good health practices is tough; even if you're the most dedicated health advocate you'll most likely have occasional slips.  However, you're kidding yourself if you think you can regularly make poor choices concerning your health and escape the consequences.  I often encounter people who tell me: *"My parents and grandparents ate high-fat diets and they all lived to their eighties." "I've smoked cigarettes for years and get fewer colds than people who have never smoked." "I don't think these doctors know what they're talking about."* There are the rare exceptions of individuals who have abused their bodies and lived long, seemingly unimpaired lives, but for most people, poor health practices take their toll.  You are a human being, not a superhuman being.

**Influences on Health**

Family and cultural influences are a deep part of your makeup, sprinkling your life with richness, uniqueness, and diversity.  However, not all of these influences are positive in regard to your health. Maria's story is one example:

*Maria was raised in an Italian home in which food played an important part. Her mother spent hours preparing dinners, and her father released stress from his hectic job in the factory by feasting on the elaborate meals.  Having lived through the Great Depression, Maria's parents viewed a plump frame as a sign of health and well-being, and encouraged their children to eat heartedly.  By the time she was in her teens, Maria was significantly obese.*

*When she went away to college, Maria learned about the principles of good nutrition and successfully shed her excess weight.  On her first visit home, her parents were critical of her slim appearance and tempted her with her past favorite foods.  When she refused the fattening treats, her mother pouted and her father accused her of "thinking she was too good for the family now that she was a college girl."*

In a family like Maria's, people may develop unhealthy eating habits because compliance with family norms yields love and acceptance.  Likewise, if as a child you observed most men stopping in the corner tavern for a few drinks each day after work and their wives merely shaking their heads when their spouses staggered home, you could become an adult who abuses or tolerates the abuse of alcohol in your own home.  The chain must be broken.

You may find yourself running in a maze of unhealthy practices.  You know you should eat fresh wholesome foods yet grabbing pizza or burgers at the local carryout is much easier. You  realize your waistline is spreading and that you're getting winded climbing stairs, yet you opt to spend your free time in front of the television rather than walking or engaging in some other form of exercise.  You see that family time has shrunk to dangerously low levels to accommodate the demands of your job, but feel you need to invest the extra time and energies in work to be competitive.  You recognize that time spent with certain relatives who are negative and critical is unpleasant and stressful yet you feel you "should" have regular contact with them.  You may continue unhealthy habits because these are quicker, easier, or more comfortable than doing what you know to be right.  Unfortunately, these habits contribute to a compromised state of health that potentially can:

- lead to a less than fully productive life
- impose burdens on others
- destroy your family
- divert your attention from God to fruitless and even sinful activities

In addition, these consequences of unhealthy habits are dishonoring to the Lord.

Perhaps you view time spent in resting, exercising, and solitude as selfish activities.  After all, how can you indulge in spending an afternoon in solitude when you could be taking the kids to the zoo?  Or, what kind of person would you be if you set limits and refused to listen to a friend who drains you with her chronic complaining while doing nothing to change the situation?  Taking care of yourself is responsible, not selfish.  If you are to follow God's command to love others as yourself you must assure you are demonstrating healthy self-love through responsible actions with your body, mind, and spirit so that you are equipped to love and serve well.

## You Do As You Believe

Your health status is influenced greatly by your beliefs---first and foremost, the belief that *God wants you to live an abundant life.* An abundant life doesn't guarantee a disease-free, painless existence; despite the most ideal practices, suffering and hardship can occur. Nor does it mean overflowing wealth so that you can buy expensive toys and enjoy a life of leisure. Rather, an abundant life in Christ is one in which you experience the fullness of a relationship with Him and are secure in the knowledge that He will provide you with what you need and the strength to flourish through suffering and hardship.

Another belief that influences your health is that *you have the ability to change unhealthy practices and develop healthy ones.* You can break the chain of unhealthy habits that you've acquired and establish a healthy lifestyle that can serve as a positive model to your friends and family. It is never too late. Some steps that can help you in changing beliefs are to:

- *Pray.* Build prayer into your daily routine. Ask the Lord to reveal those aspects of your life that are displeasing to Him and to guide you in making necessary changes. Pray for specific areas of change. (*"Lord, help me to organize my time so that I can do my exercises each day." "Father, please give me strength to resist temptation and not eat harmful foods." "Dear God, please keep my mind from wandering during my prayer time."*) Confess your shortcomings and offer praise for accomplishments. Pray with the expectation that your prayers will be answered and persist, even when you cannot see immediate results. And ask other Christians to pray for you, as well.
- *Journal.* Keep a written record of your struggles and accomplishments. Read through your entries and try to detect patterns, such as going off your diet whenever your mother-in-law visits or drinking a few beers when you've had a tough day at work. Recognize accomplishments, offer praise, and reward yourself.
- *Memorize scripture.* The wisdom written within the Bible can provide wonderful encouragement and guidance. Some useful verses could include *Show me your ways, O Lord, teach me your paths* (Psalm 25:4), *It is God who arms me with strength and makes my way perfect* (Psalm 18:32), *…you stoop down to make me great* (Psalm 18:35), *He gives strength to the weary and increases the power of the weak* (Isaiah 41:29), *Your attitude should be the same as that of Jesus Christ* (Philippians 2:5).
- *Use affirmations.* Develop a few statements that positively reflect your goal. (*"I can lose 20 pounds." "I am able to relieve my stress by taking a walk rather than having a drink." "I can complete 15 minutes of exercises every morning." "I have the Lord by my side to face this challenge."*) Replace any fear of failure with a mental script for success.

The belief that you can have a healthy, abundant life serves as a foundation for all your actions and enables you to plant the seeds of success.

> *"Don't be afraid; just believe."*
> Mark 5:36

## Study Questions

1. What warnings should Christians heed in regard to worldviews on health and health care practices?
2. How does accepting God's will differ from believing that you can't change fate in regard to your health status?
3. What influence does physical and mental health have on your spiritual state?
4. How may a person who has a disease still be considered healthy?
5. What motivates individuals to promote unhealthy practices within their families?

## Related scriptures to pray

Psalm 59:9-10
Matthew 5:3-12
      8:21-27
      14:35-36
      15:8-20
Mark 13:31
1John 2:15-17
      5:1-15
2Timothy 1:13-15

# CHAPTER 3
# ASSESS WHERE YOU ARE

So, you say that you believe you can live a healthy abundant life?   In that case, your next step is to take stock of the current state of your body, mind, and spirit.  The self assessment tool that follows reviews major aspects of your health status.  To do it justice, block out some uninterrupted time so that you can give some careful thought to your responses.  Try to answer these questions as thoroughly as possible as they will help you later when you consider habits that you can acquire to improve your health in a holistic manner.  Here it goes.

---

## *Self-Assessment of Health*

Age______  Marital status______  Children______  Occupation__________________

Height______  Current weight______  Weight range______

**Diet**

Please describe your food intake in a typical day:

*Describe all that are present:*

______Indigestion, heartburn

______Regurgitation

______Use of antacids

______Poor appetite

______Nausea, vomiting

______Chronic halitosis

Condition of teeth:

Do you fast?  If so, describe:

Nutritional supplements (Vitamins, Minerals, Herbs, Enzymes) used; give amount and type:

Please check the frequency of intake of the following foods:

| | *Daily (amount)* | *Sometimes* | *Rarely* | *Comments/Related Factors* |
|---|---|---|---|---|
| Fruit | ______ | ______ | ______ | __________________ |
| Fruit juices | ______ | ______ | ______ | __________________ |
| Vegetables | ______ | ______ | ______ | __________________ |
| Vegetable juices | ______ | ______ | ______ | __________________ |
| Red meat | ______ | ______ | ______ | __________________ |
| Poultry | ______ | ______ | ______ | __________________ |
| Fish | ______ | ______ | ______ | __________________ |
| Milk | ______ | ______ | ______ | __________________ |
| Cheese | ______ | ______ | ______ | __________________ |
| Pasta | ______ | ______ | ______ | __________________ |
| Bread, rolls | ______ | ______ | ______ | __________________ |
| Cereal | ______ | ______ | ______ | __________________ |
| Beans, peas | ______ | ______ | ______ | __________________ |
| Coffee | ______ | ______ | ______ | __________________ |
| Tea (caffeinated) | ______ | ______ | ______ | __________________ |
| Soda | ______ | ______ | ______ | __________________ |
| Candy | ______ | ______ | ______ | __________________ |

| | *Daily (amount)* | *Sometimes* | *Rarely* | *Comments / Related Factors* |
|---|---|---|---|---|
| Cakes, pies | _______ | _______ | _______ | _____________________ |
| Ice cream | _______ | _______ | _______ | _____________________ |
| Chocolate | _______ | _______ | _______ | _____________________ |
| Salty snacks | _______ | _______ | _______ | _____________________ |
| Table salts | _______ | _______ | _______ | _____________________ |
| Sugar | _______ | _______ | _______ | _____________________ |
| Sugar substitute | _______ | _______ | _______ | _____________________ |
| Beer | _______ | _______ | _______ | _____________________ |
| Wine | _______ | _______ | _______ | _____________________ |
| Hard liquor | _______ | _______ | _______ | _____________________ |
| Water | _______ | _______ | _______ | _____________________ |

## Activity

*Check if present and describe:*

______Difficulty walking or moving

______Joint pain or stiffness

______Muscle cramps, pain

______Muscles too loose, too tight

______Frequent fractures, sprains

______Brittle bones, osteoporosis

______History of falling

Type and frequency of exercise:

## Breathing and Circulation

*Check if present and describe:*

______Allergies

______Nasal stuffiness

______Chronic "running nose"

______Shortness of breath

______Cough

______Wheezing, asthma

______Frequent colds

______Chest pain

______Palpitations

______Numbness

______Dizziness, lightheadedness

______Leg cramps

______Varicose veins

______History of smoking


## Sleep Pattern

Usual bedtime______ Usual wake-up time______

Napping pattern:

Do you awaken refreshed?

Insomnia?  Describe:

Fatigue?  Describe

Sleep aids:

Quality of sleep:

Factors interrupting sleep:

## Elimination Pattern

*Check if present and describe:*

______Urination difficulty, dribbling

______Pain or burning with urination

______Voiding during night

______Inability to pass urine, hesitancy

______Incontinence

______Blood in urine

______Constipation

______Diarrhea

______Gas (flatus)

______Irritable bowel syndrome

______Blood in stool

______Hemorrhoids

______Laxative use

______Enema use, colonic irrigations


## Skin and Hair

*Check if present and describe:*

______Rashes

______Itching

______Unusual sensations

______Foul body odor

______Dry skin

______Oily skin

______Unusual marks or moles

______History of shingles

______Hair loss, breakage

______Dry scalp

______Brittle nails

______Soft nails

## Reproductive

*Check if present and describe:*

### Female

______Vaginal discharge

______Vaginal dryness

______Hysterectomy

______Problems with sexual function

______Change in sex drive, interest

______Pain during intercourse

______Breast abnormalities


Perform monthly self-exam of breasts?

Date of last mammogram:

Date of last GYN exam:

*If menopausal:*

Year began:

______Symptoms:

______Estrogen replacement therapy

*If menstruating:*

______Regular menstruation

______Painful menstruation

______PMS


### Male

______Discharge, itching of genitalia

______Erection difficulties

______Change in sex drive

______Prostate problems

______Perform testicular self-exam

______Breast swelling, abnormalities

Date of last prostate exam:

## Sensory

*Check if present and describe:*

______Wear eyeglasses

______Poor vision

______Cataracts

______Glaucoma

______See halos around lights

______Cloudy vision

______Pain in eyes

______Dry eyes

______Watery eyes

______Poor hearing

______Excess ear wax

______Unusual sensations, tingling

______Numbness

______Paralysis

______Decreased taste

______Unusual taste in mouth

______Inability to smell

______Smell unusual odors

______Sensitive to scents/odors, describe:

Date of last eye exam:                    Date of last hearing exam:


## General Symptoms

*Check if present and describe:*

______Frequent colds, infections

______Headaches

______Pain

______Unusual fatigue

______Swelling

______Other:

## Emotional and Spiritual

*Check if present and describe:*

______Depressed

______Anxious

______Moody, mood swings

______Hyperactive

______Suicidal thoughts

______Episodes of confusion

______Inability to focus

______Easily cry   ______Never cry

______Feel hopeless

______Paranoid, suspicious

______Argumentative

______Passive

______Difficulty maintaining relationships

______Marital conflict, problems

______Difficulty coping

______High level of stress in life

     Measures to manage stress:


______Belief in God, relationship with Jesus Christ

______Read Bible regularly

______Have accepted Jesus Christ as my savior

______Connection with church/ other Christians

______Feel spiritually empty, distressed

______Feel worthless

______Feel life has no meaning

Changes I would like to make in my life:

| Known Health Conditions/Diagnoses | Treatment/Management |
| --- | --- |
|  |  |

## Prescription and Nonprescription Medications Used

| Medication | Dosage | Reason Used |
| --- | --- | --- |
|  |  |  |

## Complaints

Please list major health complaints you have about your health in order of importance:

Please share any other information that you believe helpful to provide an understanding of your health status and needs:

## Landmarks in Your Life History

Often, significant events, positive and negative, can provide an understanding of your current health status and needs. Divide your life into decades and remember the significant occurrences during each decade. These can include the loss of a significant person, change in school or job, relationship started or terminated, illness of self or significant others, traumatic experiences, period of spiritual growth or distress, etc.

List the occurrences in the appropriate decade. (Use additional paper if needed).

| Age | Description of Significant Occurrence |
|---|---|
| 1-9 | |
| 10-19 | |
| 20-29 | |
| 30-39 | |
| 40-49 | |
| 50-59 | |
| 60-69 | |
| 70-79 | |
| 80+ | |

You may feel that completing this assessment was a tedious process.  Perhaps you've never had to participate in such a comprehensive assessment of your health status.  Unfortunately, the realities of our health care system are that many practitioners are too busy to spend time getting to know the minds, bodies, and spirits of their clients and insurance reimbursement favors the treatment of symptoms and diseases rather than the nurture and care of the whole person.  This presents a challenge for you to be an informed, proactive health care consumer so that you will be able to:

- understand the many influences on your health
- identify problems and relationships among your mind, body, and spirit that may not be readily apparent to your health care provider
- be able to seek the assistance you need from the source best able to help you (e.g., physician, clergy, nutritionist, counselor, etc.)

Put your self-assessment aside for now and turn your attention to some of the basic needs that all human beings share; these are:

Respiration
Food and water
Elimination of wastes
Movement and exercise
Activity
Sleep and rest
Safety
Normality
Solitude
Purpose
Connection with God, self, other people, nature

These needs seem fairly simple at first glance, but their fulfillment relies on several complex factors, including:

- *Physical, mental, and socioeconomic factors:*  A person who is paralyzed and unable to lift a utensil to her mouth or someone who has Alzheimer's disease and cannot remember what to do when food is placed before him may be able to chew, swallow, and digest food, but lack the ability to get food into his or her mouth due to physical or mental impairments.  Likewise, a senior citizen on a fixed income may omit the medications that her body needs to function normally, because she lacks adequate funds to pay for the prescription.
- *Knowledge, skills, and experience:*  A pregnant woman who is unaware that alcohol can be dangerous to her baby may continue drinking and threaten the safety of her child.  A person who lacks an understanding of the significance of a relationship with Christ may experience hopelessness and depression in an existence without spiritual meaning.
- *Desire and decision to act.*  An individual could describe the food pyramid and list foods that are harmful, yet continue to consume junk foods.  A person may know that an adulterous relationship is sinful and risks destroying his health, job, and family yet be unwilling to terminate the affair.

Go through your self-assessment and highlight or circle **signs, symptoms**, and unusual or abnormal **habits**. Now, think about the specific need that is affected by the signs and symptoms and write them under the appropriate heading in column A on the Action Plan on the next page. Some signs and symptoms can affect several needs. For example, "Use of antacids" can be listed under *Food and Water* and *Safety*; "Unusual fatigue" can be listed under *Movement and Activity, Sleep and Rest, Connection, Safety,* and *Normality.*

Now, examine the signs, symptoms, and habits and try to consider the **underlying reason(s)** that could be responsible, such as *eating a lot of fried foods* for "Use of antacids" and *eating poorly and having stressful job* for "Unusual fatigue." Jot down what you believe the underlying reason to be in column B. In some circumstances, you may not know the underlying reason; it is fine to put a question mark in the column.

Lastly, in column C, write an **action** you can take to change or reduce the sign, symptom, or habit, such as *reduce meals at fast food restaurants to once a week* or *discuss excessive workload with supervisor.* For some signs, symptoms, and habits, your action may need to be to obtain a medical evaluation, seek the counsel of clergy, or pray for insight and guidance into the situation.

Following the blank Action Plan for your use is one that shows some options to consider under each category.

Now that you've completed some honest self-examination, the next few chapters will guide you in exploring how you can maintain and improve your health.

## Your Action Plan to Improve Your Health

| Need | A<br>Sign/Symptom/Habit | B<br>Underlying Reason | C<br>Action |
|---|---|---|---|
| **Respiration** | | | |
| **Food and water** | | | |
| **Elimination of wastes** | | | |
| **Movement and activity** | | | |
| **Sleep and rest** | | | |
| **Solitude** | | | |
| **Connection with God, other people, nature** | | | |
| **Safety** | | | |
| **Normality** | | | |

## *Sample Items to Include In Your Action Plan*

| Need | A<br>Sign/Symptom/Habit | B<br>Underlying Reason | C<br>Action |
|---|---|---|---|
| **Respiration** | Chronic cough<br><br>Shortness of breath when climbing >15 stairs | Smoking<br><br>Poor physical condition | Enroll in smoking cessation plan<br>Begin exercise program<br>Do deep breathing exercises several times throughout the day |
| **Food and water** | Frequent heartburn<br><br><br>High intake of snack food | High intake of fried food<br>Eat while working-<br>→stressed mealtime<br>Don't have time to go to cafeteria at lunch time; rely on vending machine items | Eliminate fried foods<br>Increase fresh foods, broiled and baked items<br>Schedule time to eat in cafeteria<br>Keep healthy snack foods in office |
| **Elimination of wastes** | Frequent constipation | Low fiber and fluid intake<br>Low activity level | Include bran cereal at breakfast<br>Eat at least 5 fresh fruits daily<br>Eat a salad at lunch<br>Adhere to exercise program |
| **Movement and activity** | Stiff joints in morning<br><br>Difficult to walk and engage in physical activity | Lack of exercise | Get physical exam to determine safety of exercise program<br>Begin exercise program<br>Park car in farthest space from building<br>Perform yoga stretches several times each day |
| **Sleep and rest** | Poor quality of sleep<br>Awake tired, difficult to get out of bed<br><br>Nod off after meals | High consumption of caffeine<br>Spouse snores loudly<br>Consume high amount of sweets | Eliminate caffeine after 4PM<br>Suggest spouse get evaluated for snoring; sleep in separate room every other night<br>Change diet |
| **Solitude** | No time alone | Care for family 24-7<br>No money to go away or get babysitter | Negotiate with spouse to have 30 minutes each day to be relieved of childcare responsibilities<br>Awaken 30 minutes before family for personal quiet time |
| **Connection with God, self, other people, nature** | Often neglect prayer life | Allow worldly demands to take priority | Discuss with friend and ask friend to hold accountable |
| **Safety** | Take higher than recommended doses of medications for headaches<br>Overuse antacids | Fail to manage stress and eat well | Eat healthier diet<br>Practice stress management techniques daily<br>Eliminate foods triggering heartburn |
| **Normality** | Overweight<br><br>No interest in sex | High consumption of snack food<br>Tired at bedtime<br>Don't feel attractive due to weight gain | Begin weight reduction diet<br>Begin exercise program<br>Discuss concerns with spouse<br>Plan romantic weekend away with spouse |

## Study Questions

1. How can spiritual distress or unrest affect all other basic needs?
2. How can you balance taking care of your body to be a good steward of the temple the Lord has given you with preoccupation with physical health to the point of idolatry?
3. What were the purposes of the healings Christ performed?
4. In what ways do sinful lifestyles contribute to health problems?

## Related scriptures to pray

Exodus 20:4
Proverbs 21:2
Matthew 6:16-18
      7: 15-20
      15:17-20
Mark 8:1-10
Luke 11:24-26
      13:15-17
John 5:5-9
Philippians 4:19

# CHAPTER 4
# LEARN TO BE HEALTHY

You are a complex creation comprised of body, mind, and spirit. These various facets of you are inseparable; balance and harmony among them are essential for health. In the holistic circles in which I travel I come in contact with many people who are highly health-conscious by secular standards. They eat nutritious diets, keep firm muscles by exercising regularly, build stress-relieving practices into their lifestyles, and keep abreast of the latest alternative therapies. However, many have no relationship with Jesus Christ--- or any faith for that matter---and feed their spiritual hunger by flocking to hear best-selling author "mystics", seeking guidance from crystals and tarot cards, communicating with vague "spirits", or venturing to exotic places to meditate with spiritual guides. From a Biblical perspective, these individuals are not whole--- healthy---regardless of how great they look or feel.

On the other hand, strong faith will not guarantee health. I've also come in contact with a fair number of Christians who pray, attend church, serve in ministry, and are committed to a close relationship with the Lord. However, some of them are grossly overweight, have lifestyles that guarantee high levels of stress, or are so involved with their ministries that they have little time left for exercise, solitude, or quality family time. They miss the mark, as well. Faith in the Lord doesn't mean you can neglect or abuse your body and mind; in fact, this can be dishonoring to Him. There must be concern for the whole---body, mind, and spirit.

Jesus Christ demonstrated concern for the whole. He tended to people's spirits so that they would know, follow, and obey him. He satisfied their spiritual hunger with the living bread that would provide eternal life. But He didn't stop there. He healed persons of diseases and disabilities, in addition to healing their souls. He showed concern for physical needs as He multiplied bread and fish to feed thousands. He comforted people during times of trouble and offered hope and encouragement. He addressed the many facets of a full life by teaching people about prayer, fasting, simplicity, solitude, submission, service, meditation, and celebration.

It is important to understand that *health is about balance---not perfection.*  You needn't look like a model, possess the mental prowess of a rocket scientist, or engage in prayer all of your waking hours to be healthy.  But, you do need to respect and care for your total being---body, mind, and spirit--- so that you can become whole.

The journey to wholeness is not without sacrifice and challenges.  And, it doesn't mean that you will be free from aches, pains, and diseases.  Health---wholeness---is possible in the presence of adversity, imperfection, and illness when you view these obstacles as purposeful challenges and opportunities for growth.  You need only examine the story of Job to see a profound example of a man who suffered through adversity and grew whole and closer to God as a result.

The remainder of this section reviews some basic health principles to assure you have a factual foundation upon which to build your health plan.  Specific topics that are covered in an effort to address whole-person care from a Christian perspective include:  *diet, elimination, movement and exercise, sleep and rest, safety (including the safe use of complementary and alternative therapies), normality, sexuality, health screening, solitude, purpose,* and *connection.* (As there are volumes written on each of these topics, you can visit your library or bookstore to explore any of them in more depth.)   As you learn about healthy lifestyle practices, understand that one approach is not right for all.  Plans for optimum health must be individualized and fully integrated---body, mind, and spirit.

**Diet**

It seems that half the population is talking about the latest diet craze and the other half about the newest restaurant or recipe they've found.  Food is a hot topic of interest and certainly has more significance than merely providing nourishment for the body.  Learning the significance of food to you is a good starting point in building good dietary practices as this can help you to identify patterns that may need to be changed.  My own eating habits can demonstrate this.  Like many people, when I'm traveling and eating in restaurants, my diet tends to reflect many items that I wouldn't regularly eat at home.  This posed no major problem for me until my work caused me to travel frequently.  As I hurried from one terminal to another to meet a tight plane connection it was easier to grab a double-dipped ice cream cone on route than to find and consume something more nutritious.  When I finally arrived at the hotel, a bacon cheeseburger (at least a quarter-pounder) and fries were much more comforting than a broiled chicken breast and broccoli.  And of course, when local acquaintances asked me to accompany them to the best restaurants in the area, I *had* to sample the special delicacies which had a tendency to be high in fat and calories.  If this had happened once in awhile it would have been manageable, but when I was out of town weekly, my exceptions to a nutritious diet were becoming routine.  Something had to change.  I now try to pack nutritious snacks in my carry-on bag so that I can avoid fast food pick-me-ups and discipline myself to select from restaurants' lower fat menu items.  Do I ever slip?  You bet!  But straying from the path of good eating even a third of the time still beats the unhealthy food consumption that was typical for me nearly every time I ate out while away from home in the past.

What influences your eating?  Do you look to food as a means of comfort and relaxation like I did when I was traveling?  Is eating a source of entertainment or a means of showing and receiving love?  Do you follow strict practices to prevent or manage a health condition?  Are you among the small minority who give little attention to eating and consume only enough to survive?

After you do some honest self-evaluation and identify behaviors that you need to change, your next step is to make sure you consume the correct diet.  Your body needs proper nourishment to function normally, grow, repair damaged tissue, reproduce, protect itself from infection and disease, and have ample energy to participate in the usual activities of daily living.  Good nutrition means that the quality and quantity of your food intake is adequate to meet your body's needs.  Excesses or deficiencies in nutrients can contribute to poor health.

Nutrition facts aren't exactly the type of material that make for interesting reading, yet you need to have a basic understanding of them to make sensible, healthy choices.  With that in mind, read through the next few pages to get a crash course on nutrients.  Try to get a general understanding of the main points and return to this section in the future when you have specific questions.

The various nutrients needed to keep the body in balance can be categorized by *macronutrients* and *micronutrients*.  Macronutrients consist of:

- *Carbohydrates* that are the main source of energy for the body and help with digestion and metabolism of proteins and fats.  They can take the form of simple carbohydrates that come from sources like table sugars and fruits, or complex carbohydrates that are provided by foods like potatoes, rice, and cereals.  A high intake of complex carbohydrates and a low intake of simple carbohydrates are recommended.
- *Proteins* that build, repair, and maintain body tissue, produce antibodies, regulate the body's acid-base balance, and detoxify harmful substances.  They are large complex molecules made of amino acids that each have a specific function.  A complete protein contains all of the amino acids; meat, eggs, and dairy products are examples of complete proteins.  Nuts, grains, and legumes are examples of incomplete proteins; they must be combined in certain ways or with a complete protein to provide a balanced amount of amino acids.
- *Fats* that are concentrated forms of heat and energy.  Different classifications of fats have different functions, such as to help to synthesize essential compounds in the body and control body temperature.  Sources of fats are whole-milk products, meats, eggs, nuts, peanut butter, olives, avocados, and vegetable oils.

Attached to macronutrients are micronutrients which consist of *vitamins* and *minerals*.  Vitamins aid in metabolism and in releasing energy from digested food.  Along with enzymes, vitamins act as catalysts in chemical reactions within the body.  Minerals help in the formation and maintenance of body fluids, blood, bone, and the nervous system. A description of common  vitamins and minerals is offered in Table 1.

## Table 1  Vitamins and Minerals

## Fat Soluble Vitamins

| Vitamin | Function | Source |
| --- | --- | --- |
| Vitamin A (Retinol) | Antioxidant.  Promotes nonspecific resistance to infection, aids in production of lysozymes in tears, saliva and sweat that help fight bacteria, stimulates cell-mediated and humoral immunity, promotes good vision and healthy tissue and hair.  Beta-carotene metabolizes into vitamin A in the body and is a stronger antioxidant than vitamin A; at least 15mg of beta-carotene daily is recommended. | Milk, butter, liver, green and yellow vegetables |
| Vitamin D | Promotes strong bones and teeth, calcium-phosphorus metabolism | Sunlight, egg yolk, organ meats, fish |
| Vitamin E | Antioxidant properties that aid in the prevention of free-radicals, enhances antibody production, maintains circulatory system; stronger immune-boosting effect when taken with selenium | Dark green vegetables, eggs, liver, wheat germ, vegetable oil, oatmeal, peanuts, tomatoes |
| Vitamin F (Unsaturated fatty acids) | Promotes healthy skin, blood coagulation, cholesterol, glandular activity | Sunflower seeds, vegetable oils |
| Vitamin K (Menadione) | Blood clotting | Green leafy vegetables, yogurt, molasses |

## Water Soluble Vitamins

| Vitamin | Function | Source |
|---|---|---|
| Vitamin B1 (Thiamin) | Promotes resistance to infection, primary immunoglobulin response, digestion, cardiovascular function, energy production | Peas, lima beans, asparagus, corn,. potatoes, blackstrap molasses, brown rice, meat, nuts, poultry, wheat germ |
| Vitamin B2 (Riboflavin) | Along with other B-complex vitamins, helps to maintain mucosal barriers that protect against infection, aids in production of antibodies and red blood cells, skin repair | Brewer's yeast, broccoli, spinach, asparagus, Brussels sprouts, peas, corn, blackstrap molasses, nuts, organ meats, whole grains |
| Vitamin B6 (Pyridoxine) | Promotes health of mucous membranes and blood vessels, involved in antibody formation, red blood cells, affects immune function more than other B-vitamins | Bananas, avocados, carrots, kale, spinach, sweet potatoes, apples, wheat germ, grains |
| Vitamin B12 (Colalamin) | Development of red blood cells, maintenance of nervous system, believed to exert regulatory influence on T-helper and suppressor cells | Cheese, fish, milk, milk products, organ meats, eggs |
| Niacin (Niacinamide B3) | Convert food to energy, healthy skin, nervous system, cell metabolism | Cereals, yeast, lean meat, liver, eggs |
| Biotin (Vitamin H) | Metabolism of protein, carbohydrates, and fats, healthy skin and circulatory system | Egg yolk, green leafy vegetables, milk, organ meats |
| Vitamin C (Ascorbic acid) | Antioxidant, wound healing, healthy gums, believed to promote phagocytic function, believed to aid in preventing common cold and influenza | Citrus fruits, berries, green peppers, broccoli, Brussels sprouts, spinach |
| Folic acid (Folacin, Folate, Vitamin B9) | Production of red blood cells, enhance immune system, normal growth | Green leafy vegetables, milk and other dairy products, organ meats, oysters, salmon, Brewer's yeast, dates, tuna, whole grains |

| Vitamin | Function | Source |
| --- | --- | --- |
| Pantothenic acid | Enhances immune system, promotes antibody formation, helps convert proteins, carbohydrates, and fats into energy | Brewer's yeast, legumes, organ meats, salmon, wheat germ, whole grains, mushrooms |
| Choline (Lecithin) | Regulates liver and gallbladder, cell membrane structure, nerve transmission | Yeast, eggs, fish, lecithin, wheat germ, organ meats, soy |
| Inositol | Metabolism of fat and cholesterol, nerve function | Molasses, yeast, lecithin, fruits, meat, milk, nuts |
| Para-aminobenzoic acid (PABA) | Pigmentation of skin, maintenance of hair color, health of blood vessel wall | Molasses, eggs, liver, milk, rice, yeast, wheat germ, bran |
| Vitamin P (Bioflavoids) | Maintenance of blood vessel wall | Skin and pulp of fruits |

## Minerals

| Mineral | Function | Source |
|---|---|---|
| Calcium | Growth and maintenance of teeth and bones, muscle contractions, nerve transmission | Milk, cheese, green vegetables |
| Chromium | Carbohydrate metabolism, energy production, glucose utilization | Yeast, whole grains, vegetable oils |
| Copper | Hemoglobin production, enzyme activity, protection from infection | Nuts, seeds, organ meats, raisins, molasses, seafood |
| Iodine | Production of thyroid hormone, regulation of metabolism | Seafood, kelp, iodized salt |
| Iron | Transport oxygen to tissues, enzyme activity, immune function | Spinach, lima beans, peas, Brussels sprouts, broccoli, strawberries, asparagus, blackstrap molasses, eggs, fish poultry, wheat germ, shredded wheat |
| Magnesium | Enzyme activity, regulation of acid-base balance, glucose metabolism, nerve function, protein production | Honey, bran, green vegetables, nuts, seafood, spinach, kelp |
| Manganese | Enzyme activity in reproduction, growth, fat metabolism | Whole grains, eggs, nuts, green vegetables |
| Phosphorus | Formation of bones and teeth, muscle contraction, kidney function, nerve and muscle activity | Eggs, fish, meat, poultry, grains, cheese |
| Potassium | Fluid-electrolyte balance, pH balance of blood, nerve and muscle function | Dates, raisins, figs, peaches, sunflower seeds |
| Selenium | Antioxidant (with vitamin E), protects cell membrane, promotes humoral immunity, potentiates activity of phagocytes | Butter, wheat germ, whole grains, seafood, eggs, brown rice, apple cider, vinegar, garlic |
| Zinc | Stimulates T cell immunity (but decreases phagocytic immunity), wound healing, development and growth of reproductive organs, production of male hormone | Brewer's yeast, liver, seafood, soybeans, spinach, sunflower seeds, mushrooms |

All nutrients are important to your body, but it is important to assure the right balance of their consumption. The MyPlate shown in Figure 1 shows the recommended daily consumption of various nutrients. As you can see, a healthy diet is rich in grains, fruits, and vegetables and limited in fats and refined and processed sugars and starches.

---

**Figure 1  MyPlate**

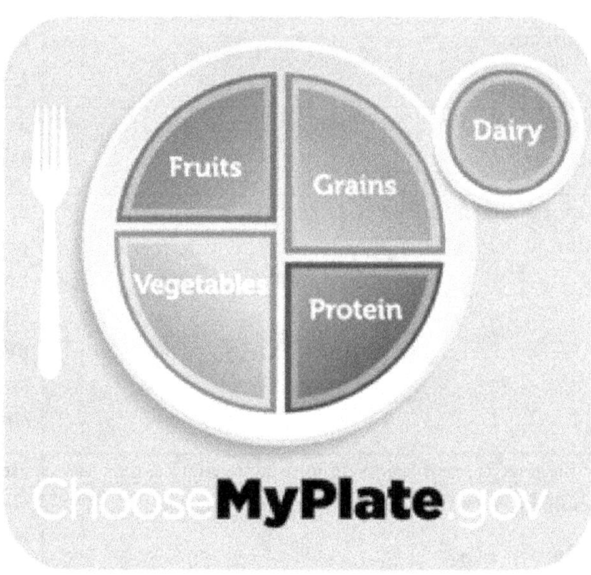


MyPlate shows the five food groups that are necessary for a healthy diet. It was developed by the U.S. Department of Agriculture. More information about MyPlate and healthy eating patterns can be obtained at https://www.choosemyplate.gov/MyPlate

---

In some circles, vegetarianism is promoted as God's desired diet plan. This belief stems from Genesis 1:29 when God said *"I give you every seed-bearing plant on the face of the whole earth and every tree that has fruit with seed in it. They will be yours for food."* While a vegetarian diet is a healthy eating plan, a purely plant-based diet is not supported by Scripture. A little farther along in Genesis 4, Abel is identified as a shepherd who gained favor by offering God the firstborn of his flock (4:4) and later (9:3) God tells Noah *"Everything that lives and moves will be food for you. Just as I gave you green plants, I now give you everything."* Jesus not only ate food other than vegetables and fruits, but also offered it to those He loved. For instance, He multiplied bread and fish to feed thousands of people for whom He felt compassion (Matthew 14:13-21, 15:32-37). Jesus was quite clear about the freedom of dietary restrictions when He clarified for His disciples that it isn't what enters a man from the outside that makes him unclean but what comes out of a man's heart (Mark 7:18-20). Jesus was more concerned with setting us free and helping us to achieve eternal life than in placing us in bondage with laws.

Although Christians are not compelled to follow dietary restrictions, the Bible is clear about dietary excesses. Gluttony is an overindulgence which is sinful. Paul describes self-control as a fruit of the spirit (Galatians 5:23), therefore, restraint in dietary practices is a virtue to be nurtured. (Obesity is discussed in greater detail in the next chapter.)

Good fluid intake is essential to health. If you did nothing but lie still all day, your body would still lose 64-80 ounces of water through fluids lost through breathing, perspiring, voiding, and bowel elimination. If you live in a dry environment or have an active lifestyle, your fluid loss is greater. To maintain fluid balance you need to consume at least the amount of fluids that your body loses, which for the average individual is six to eight 8-ounce glasses of fluids daily. Most of your fluid intake should be in the form of plain water. While coffee, tea, sodas, and alcoholic beverages do contain water, they also contain substances that can increase fluid loss and threaten your body's health, so limit their intake.

## Elimination

Although not a popular topic of social conversation, eliminating wastes from the body is crucial to health. Wastes from your tissues are carried in the blood to the kidneys where they are filtered and excreted in urine. A good fluid intake assists in removing these waste products.

Bowel elimination tends to be a greater problem for most people than urinary elimination, evidenced by laxative sales in this country. Often, irregularity in bowel elimination is the result of diet or inactivity. In addition to some exercise, bowel elimination can be promoted by:

- Eating a high-fiber diet
- Reducing the consumption of processed foods
- Drinking several glasses of juice daily
- Providing adequate time for toileting

If constipation is a problem, natural measures rather than medications can be used as a first line of attack to help stimulate bowel movements. Vitamin C supplements (not to exceed 2000 mg per day) can help to soften stools, as well as herbs like dandelion root, cascara sagrada, and senna that can be used for their laxative effect.

You need only examine the labels of popular foods to see that a variety of chemicals are ingested through the average American diet. These chemicals can cause toxins to accumulate in the body and threaten your health. Elimination of these toxins is helpful and fasting is a beneficial means of accomplishing this. You may want to plan an occasional fast, such as one day each month. (The next chapter discusses fasting in greater detail to guide you through this process.)

## Movement and Exercise

Movement involves changing from one position or place to another. Your internal body is in a constant state of motion, witnessed by the circulation of blood through your vessels, the exchange of air in your lungs, the passage of food through your digestive tract, and the blinking of your eyes. Some of the movements you make, such as walking, are the result of voluntary effort on your part. Others, such as the secretion of hormones and the filtration of wastes through the kidneys, occur without you consciously having to think about them. God's creative capacity certainly is evidenced in these purposeful, efficient, and complex activities of the human body. Movement and exercise of the body have numerous benefits (see Table 2). You will need to tailor an exercise program to your individual needs. Before embarking on any exercise program, be sure to have a physical examination so that you'll be aware of any precautions you must heed. For instance, some heart and blood pressure medications can alter your heart's response to exercise, demanding that some adjustments be made. (Specific guidelines regarding exercise are offered in the next chapter.)

You may believe that you are getting ample exercise because you are on the go throughout the day. Actually, you can be physically active to the point of exhaustion but not truly exercising. Exercise is the conscious act of moving in order to maintain strength or function. There are different types of exercises, including:

- *Strengthening:* exercises that should be done every other day to develop and improve muscle tone, such as weight training, playing tennis, and performing physical labor
- *Aerobic:* exercises that involve activities such as brisk walking, bicycling, jumping rope, and swimming that are helpful to do at least several times during the week
- *Flexibility:* gentle stretching, such as tai chi or yoga, that are useful to do daily

---

### Table 2  Benefits of Exercise

Improves circulation
Strengthens immune system
Aids in reducing weight and body fat
Increases bone density and strength
Keeps muscles strong and in tone
Reduces blood pressure
Increases lung capacity and air exchange
Increases insulin sensitivity and glucose tolerance
Promotes regular bowel elimination
Reduces risk of some cancers
Elevates mood
Increases energy
Improves mental function
Promotes restful sleep
Relieves stress

*Exercise of Spiritual Disciplines*

In addition to physical training, the exercise of the spiritual disciplines is important to enable your life to bear fruit. Just as you move your body in a conscious manner to maintain and strengthen your physical health, consciously developing your spirit will help you to maintain and strengthen your relationship with the Lord. The spiritual disciplines include meditation, prayer, fasting, study, simplicity, solitude, submission, service, confession, worship, guidance, and celebration[1]. These spiritual practices are as essential to a vital state of holistic health as eating, therefore, they cannot be omitted from any discussion of a healthy lifestyle. (The spiritual disciplines will be discussed in more detail later.)

## Sleep and Rest

> *...so on the seventh day He rested from all his work.* Genesis 2:2
> *Come with me by yourselves to a quiet place and get some rest.* Mark 6:31

Your creator appreciated the value of rest to the extent that He could put aside His work for a day. Likewise, Jesus showed His understanding of the need for rest when He urged the disciples to rest so that they would be refreshed and renewed to effectively minister. You must question what, by comparison, do *you* do that is so important that it warrants shortchanging your sleep and rest?

Periods of rest and sleep are essential to refresh and renew the body, mind, and spirit. They help you to maintain balance and a sense of well-being.

Sleep is controlled by two specialized areas of the brain:
*Reticular activating system (RAS)* which is associated with wakefulness
*Bulbar synchronizing region (BSR)* which is most active during sleep
These two systems are thought to intermittently activate and then suppress the brain centers causing periods of wakefulness and sleep.

There are two kinds of sleep: *rapid eye movement (REM)* and *non-rapid eye movement or slow wave (NREM) sleep*. A normal sleep cycle consists of four stages of NREM and a final stage of REM sleep (Table 3).

Rest is a period of inactivity and peace. A period of inactivity doesn't necessarily mean you are resting. (If you've ever laid in bed in the middle of the night thinking about something you needed to do the following day you understand this!) Peace of mind promotes rest and sleep. God wants you to have peace of mind and invites you to pray and petition him for this. *Do not be anxious about anything, but in everything, by prayer and petition, with thanksgiving, present your requests to God* (Philippians 4:6). Have sufficient faith in God to turn your worries over to him.

Some practical hints for promoting rest and sleep are offered in the next chapter.

## Table 3 Stages of Sleep

*Stage I NREM (Non-Rapid Eye Movement)*
- Light sleep from which sleeper can be easily awakened
- Eyes roll from side to side
- Heart and respiratory rates slightly decrease
- Advances to next stage within several minutes if no disturbance
- Sleep interrupted during any other stage will cause cycle to return to Stage I

*Stage II NREM Sleep*
- Continued light sleep with higher state of relaxation
- Sleep remains light and easily broken
- Continued decline in temperature and heart and respiratory rates
- Eyes are still

*Stage III NREM Sleep*
- Early stage of deep sleep
- Continued slowing of bodily processes
- Relaxation of muscles
- Moderate stimulation required to arouse sleeper

*Stage IV NREM Sleep*
- Extreme relaxation, deepest stage of sleep usually reached in 20-30 minutes and lasting about 30 minutes
- Decreased vital signs and body movements
- Considerable stimulation required to arouse sleeper
- This stage diminished with age and may be absent in some older adults
- It is believed that this stage is essential to physically restoring the body

*REM (Rapid Eye Movement) Sleep*
- Most dreaming and sleep talking occur
- Decreased tonus of head and neck muscles
- Increase and possibly irregularity of heart beat and respirations
- Electroencephalogram (EEG) resembles Stage I
- Sleepers drift into REM from Stage IV about once every 90 minutes, four to five times each night
- Can be disrupted by amphetamines, alcohol, barbiturates, or phenothiazine derivatives
- Deprivation can result in irritability, anxiety, acute psychotic episodes

## Safety

Air pollution…crime…terrorists…tainted meats…tornadoes…. The world is full of hazards, many of which are beyond your control.  However, there are threats to your health and well-being that you can protect yourself against.

Your first lines of defense is to keep yourself healthy.  Many of the measures already discussed, such as good nutrition, adequate rest, and regular exercise contribute to your health and can assist in giving you resistance against illness.

Boosting your immunity is an important measure and far surpasses treating infections and diseases after they have invaded your body.  If you have a chronic health problem, such as emphysema or diabetes, or if you are an older adult, you have a higher than normal risk for developing infections and need to actively prevent them by strengthening your immunity.  Table 4 lists some ways in which you can enhance the function of your immune system.  In addition, be careful not to overuse antibiotics.  Overuse of antibiotics can disrupt the body's natural balance and enable new infections to develop (as women who have developed vaginal infections after using antibiotics can attest).  Excess antibiotic use can cause bacteria to become resistant to these drugs, also.

---

### Table 4  Strengthening the Immune System

*Diet:*  milk, yogurt, nonfat cottage cheese, eggs, fresh fruits and vegetables, grains, nuts, onion, sprouts, pure honey, unsulfured molasses
*Herbs:*  echinacea, goldenseal, ginseng, garlic
*Exercise:*  any form of moderate regular exercise
*Stress management:*  meditation, progressive relaxation, periods of solitude
*Attitude:*  open, assertive, trusting, altruistic, loving, appreciative

---

*Safe Use of Complementary and Alternative Therapies*

There has been an explosion in the use of herbal remedies, acupuncture, chiropractic, magnet therapy, and other complementary and alternative therapies.  Complementary and alternative therapies are those health promotion and healing practices that fall outside the realm of conventional medical practice in our country (Table 5).  Nearly half of all Americans use some form of complementary and alternative medicine, spending billions of dollars annually.  The National Institutes of Health has created a National Center for Complementary and Integrative Health to support research and integration of these therapies into the conventional health care system.  Andrew Weil, Deepak Chopra, and other gurus of alternative medicine are prominent in the media.

There have been legitimate reasons for the skyrocketing interest in complementary and alternative therapies.  Experiences with mainstream medical care have left much to be desired as five minute impersonal office visits have replaced the warm relationship shared with the old family doctor. Alternative therapists who invest time to learn about and listen to their clients have offered positive experiences to consumers. Many people want to use natural approaches to treat illnesses and avoid using medications and other interventions that carry high risks for complications. Americans have become aware of interesting and new healing techniques as communication and knowledge of other cultural practices have increased. Physicians, nurses, and other conventional health care professionals are integrating complementary and alternative therapies into their practices and teaching these therapies in their schools.

The popularity of complementary and alternative therapies assures that Christians will encounter them and consider their use. Discernment is essential as choices are made. Just because a therapy has been used for centuries or is promoted by a charismatic leader doesn't make it effective. Some therapies are based on the beliefs or testimonies of a small minority of people; research may be nonexistent or limited to sample sizes too small to have results be significant. The fact that a substance is "natural" doesn't mean it cannot cause harmful effects. An example is the herb gingko biloba that many people use for memory enhancement that can thin the blood and cause serious bleeding problems in some people. Some alternative therapists may be skilled in practicing their specific modality but lack comprehensive education that could enable them to properly recognize a wide range of health conditions; conditions may go undiagnosed and treatment delayed as a result.

A major consideration for Christians in the use of alternative therapies is that some are based on Eastern, New Age, or other faiths that are in conflict with Christianity. These practices go against Biblical teachings and rely on sources of spiritual intervention other than Jesus Christ. Table 5 describes some popular complementary and alternative therapies and how they could pose a problem for Christians. Table 6 provides some tips for discerning these therapies.

**Table 5**

**Popular Complementary and Alternative Therapies and Related Concerns**

| Therapy | Description | Concerns |
|---|---|---|
| **Acupuncture/ Acupressure** | Based on principles of traditional Chinese medicine, these systems are based on the theory that the body has invisible energy channels known as meridians. *Chi*, or life energy is thought to run through these meridians. Blockages or imbalances of chi can cause symptoms. By inserting needles (acupuncture) or applying pressure (acupressure) at specific points along the meridians energy flow can be unblocked. | Acupuncturists must complete special training and in most states be licensed. Treatments by an unskilled or careless practitioner could result in infection or injury.<br><br>Some practitioners may integrate Eastern religions or call on spiritual powers with their practice and these could conflict with Christianity. |
| **Ayurveda** | Traditional medicine of India that places equal emphasis on body, mind, and spirit. Based on theory that life is sustained by invisible life energy called *prana* and that individuals have different metabolic body types, *doshas*. When the dosha is out of balance, illness occurs. Uses herbs, yoga, diet, meditation, detoxification, massage, breathing exercises, mental hygiene, spiritual healing, and exposure to sunlight. | Worldviews that conflict with Christianity are used (e.g., Transcendental Meditation to achieve altered states of consciousness, Hinduism overtones). Inclusion of spiritual healing in this system lends itself to practitioner suggesting or imposing non-Christians beliefs. |
| **Biofeedback** | System of learning to bring certain bodily functions (such as heart rate, blood pressure, temperature) under voluntary control. Usually an electronic device initially is used to provide feedback of body responses. Eventually, people learn ways to elicit response without use of machine. Not based on any spiritual beliefs or faith systems. | Low risk. |
| **Chiropracty** | Specialty that uses manipulation or adjustment of spine and joints to restore alignment. Based on belief that misalignments can cause altered body function and symptoms. Popularly used for treatment of back problems. | Injuries can occur with unskilled practitioner.<br><br>Some chiropractors may incorporate New Age or other approaches that are not consistent with Christianity. |

| Therapy | Description | Concerns |
|---|---|---|
| **Herbal Therapies** | Use of various parts of plants for medicinal reasons. Can be used internally or externally. | Although natural substances, herbs are not without their risks. They can cause serious adverse effects and interact with drugs.<br><br>To assure safety and standardized dose, need to be obtained from reliable sources. |
| **Homeopathy** | Homeopathic remedies are dilute forms of biological materials (plants, minerals, etc) that produce symptoms similar to that caused by disease. An extract of the substance is made and diluted many times. The more dilute a substance is, the higher its potency. The solution is then added to a sugar tablet, ointment, or other substance. | Low risk.<br><br>Although remedies can be purchased over the counter, ideal approach is to have homeopath compound remedy based on individual profile and symptoms.<br><br>Many positive anecdotal reports although research is inconclusive as to effectiveness. |
| **Iridology** | Examination of eye's iris to diagnose health problems. Based on belief that diseases create visible patterns in different parts of the iris. Different parts of the iris represent different parts of the body. | Low risk although no scientific evidence supporting it.<br><br>Practitioner may offer products for sale to treat alleged conditions discovered during exam. |
| **Magnetic Therapies** | Based on belief that magnets have healing powers due to ability to improve circulation and stimulate nerve endings. | Low risk although should not be used in persons with a pacemaker, who have cancer, or who are pregnant.<br><br>Some evidence that they could be useful for pain management; little evidence for other benefits. |
| **Meditation** | An activity that calms the mind and promotes relaxation. Can include focusing on breathing, sensations, or specific thoughts; visualizing an image; repeating a word or chant. | If mind focuses is on power other than God or biblical truths, the mind can be left open to non-Christian spiritual influences.<br><br>Psychological problems can arise in vulnerable individuals. |
| **Naturopathy** | System of health care that uses good health practices and natural means to prevent and care for illness. Emphasize a holistic approach. | Low risk.<br><br>Some doctors of naturopathy may promote New Age approaches to health and spirituality, although this is not an essential framework for this practice. |

| Therapy | Description | Concerns |
|---|---|---|
| **Nutritional Supplements** | Use of vitamins, minerals, and other nutrients to improve general health and address specific health concerns. | Excess doses of some supplements can be harmful and cause life-threatening effects. Advisable not to exceed recommended dosage range without professional supervision. |
| **Qigong** | Practice within system of traditional Chinese medicine consisting of meditation, breathing exercises, and repetitive movements.  Aims to unify person with universal life energy.  Used for relaxation, stress management, and to promote general well-being. | Practitioners may claim that Qigong can cure illnesses whereas there is no evidence to support this.<br><br>Life energy that practice is supposed to connect one with may not be God; other religious beliefs could serve as foundation. |
| **Reflexology** | Based on theory that areas of the foot and hand correspond to body organs; massage and pressure to these areas can relieve symptoms in the corresponding organ. | Low risk.<br><br>Few controlled studies to support claims.<br><br>Some reflexologists may promote Eastern religious beliefs if they consider their actions to be affected universal life energy. |
| **Reiki** | Practice of improving flow of life energy by practitioner placing hands on or over 12 different locations and serving as conduit to allow energy to transfer through. Various sensations may be felt by the recipient. | Few controlled studies to support claims.<br><br>Practitioners could communicate with and draw their energy from spiritual sources other than God. |
| **Tai chi** | Exercise consisting of meditation, breathing exercises, and slow graceful movements.  Within traditional Chinese medicine, tai chi is believed to enhance and balance the flow of chi. | Low risk.<br><br>. |
| **Therapeutic Touch** | Practice whereby practitioner pass hands over a person's body, several inches from the surface, to manipulate the energy field for the promotion of health and treatment of various health conditions. | Has Eastern mysticism underpinnings which are not compatible with Christianity.<br><br>Research is conflicting on effectiveness and claimed benefits. |

---

**Table 6  Checklist for Discerning Complementary and Alternative Modalities (CAM)**

___ You have obtained a conventional physical exam to understand your health state
   prior to using CAM.

___ Scientific evidence exists supporting the claims made by the selected CAM.

___ The CAM practitioner works in concert with conventional medical practitioners and refers to
   them when needed.

___ The CAM practitioner doesn't claim that he or she possesses special healing powers and doesn't call on
   special spirits for healing.

___ The CAM does not require that other religious systems be supported or practiced.

___ The CAM practitioner is licensed or certified as required by the state.

___ The CAM practice or product is not in conflict with biblical doctrine.

___ The CAM product is labeled and standardized.

___ Claims of the CAM practitioner can be validated by another source.

___ The CAM practitioner allows you to purchase prescribed products from any source
   and does not require you purchase only from him/her

---

## Normality

An important aspect of health involves keeping your body makeup and function within normal limits. This includes such things as assuring you have a blood pressure below 140/90, a regular heart beat, unobstructed blood circulation, and blood chemistry within a normal range. Good health practices and prompt attention to symptoms of health problems assist in maintaining normality.

### *Sexuality*

The norms for sexuality and sexual function have been tested and stretched to the point that our society conveys the message that sexual normality is an individual determination:  there is no right or wrong, nor normal or abnormal.  Interestingly, as acceptance of any type of sexual expression has increased, so have the rates of children born into single-parent homes, teen pregnancies, divorce, and sexually-transmitted diseases. Christians need only to visit the Bible  to gain insight into God's expectations regarding normal sexual function.  For instance:

- *Do you not know that your body is a temple of the Holy Spirit, who is in you, whom you have received from God? You are not your own; you were bought at a price.  Therefore, honor God with you body.* 1 Corinthians 6:19-20
- *It is God's will that you should be sanctified; that you should avoid sexual immorality; that each of you should learn to control his own body in a way that is holy and honorable…* 1 Thessalonians 4:3
- *You shall not commit adultery.* Exodus 20:14
- *You must not bring the earnings of a female prostitute or of a male prostitute into the house of the Lord your God to pay any vow, because the Lord your God detests them both.* Deuteronomy 23:18
- *The husband should fulfill his marital duty to his own wife, and each woman her husband.* 1 Corinthians 7:3

- *Do not deprive each other except by mutual consent and for a short time, so that you may devote yourselves to prayer. Then come together again so that Satan will not tempt you because of your lack of self-control.*  1 Corinthians 7:5
- *If a man has sexual relations with an animal, he must be put to death, and you must kill the animal.  If a woman approaches an animal to have sexual relations with it, kill both the woman and the animal.*  Leviticus 20:15-16
- *If a man marries his sister, the daughter of either his father or his mother, and they have sexual relations, it is a disgrace.*  Leviticus 20:17
- *Flee from sexual immorality.*  1 Corinthians 6:18

God established these norms of sexual behavior because He created the sanctity of marriage and the family, and wanted to protect you from the disease, pain, and turmoil that results from sexual sins.  Honoring these norms demonstrates your love and obedience to the Lord and promotes a healthy, balanced, life.

*Health Screening*

In order to maintain normality, you need to be able to identify abnormalities.  Sometimes, signs and symptoms alert you to the fact that something is wrong, as what occurs when you experience a fever, find a lump on your body, or notice a significant change in your mood.  However, there are many abnormalities that you cannot detect in an early stage and that require special types of examinations and tests in order to be detected.  Regular, comprehensive physical check-ups can aid in detecting health conditions early, and some of the specific tests and exams that are important to include are:

- Blood pressure reading
  - Preferably annually, but at least every two years if your blood pressure is less than 120/80 mm Hg
  - As your health provider recommends, but at least every year if your blood pressure ranges from 120 to 139 mm Hg for the top number (systolic), or 80 to 89 mm Hg for the bottom number (diastolic)
- Cholesterol screening
  - Starting at age 20, every 5 years; if results abnormal, more frequent screening is recommended
- Diabetes screening
  - After age 45 every 3 years; if obese or other risk factors are present, screening may begin earlier
- Colon and rectal cancer screening
  - Starting at age 50, or at age 45 if you're African-American. Consider earlier screening if at high risk of colon cancer or rectal cancer (e.g., due to personal or family history of colon or rectal cancer or polyps or inflammatory bowel disease)
- Gynecological (GYN) exam
  - Pap test every two years. If you've had three normal Pap tests in a row, you may need a Pap test only once every three years. You may be able to stop Pap tests between ages 65 and 70 if you've had three normal Pap tests in a row and no abnormal test results in the past 10 years. You may also be able to stop Pap tests if you've had a hysterectomy with removal of the cervix.
- Mammogram for women
  - At age 40 every 1-2 years; yearly after age 50

    o    Women under age 40 should have clinical breast exams by a health care provider at least every 3 years; mammograms may be recommended based on risk.

In addition, you can aid in detecting health problems early by performing self-examinations of your breast if you're a woman and self-examination of testes if you're a man. Your health care provider can explain the procedures for these self-examinations to you and you also can obtain information from your local chapter of the American Cancer Society. Be sure to have any abnormality that you note evaluated as early as possible.

## Solitude

*"Dad, remember that you have to drive me and the guys to school today" shouted Doug's son from the hallway. Not only had he not remembered, but Doug realized that he also had a few extra phone calls to make prior to going to his office this morning. With a coffee mug, briefcase, and three teenage boys in tow, Doug raced from the house. The boys' chatter dashed any hopes of being able to make any phone calls from the car until the stop at school.*

*Doug had barely pulled out of the school lot when his cell phone rang. He recognized his associate's number and promptly pulled out his cell phone to learn what the problem was. After two more phone calls and miles of rush hour traffic, Doug finally reached the office. He checked his voice mail messages while removing his coat and realized two calls needed to be made before entering his meeting. Fortunately, the 21 emails consisted of nothing that couldn't wait until later. As he walked to the meeting he was joined by a few coworkers who wanted to chat about the new vacation policy that had been posted.*

*After a morning-long intense meeting, Doug decided to go out for lunch to get his mind clear. He found lines at the first two restaurants he went to so he opted for a soda and hot dog from a street vendor. The only free seat Doug could find in the park was an end of a bench which also was occupied by a couple in the midst of a heated argument. He gulped down his lunch and weaved through the crowds to return to his office for an afternoon of more of the same.*

Your days may be similar to Doug's in that you often are engaged in some activity from the time you awaken until the time you lay your head on the pillow; even then your brain may be racing with thoughts of things you have to do, people you need to see. Voice mails, cell phones, emails, faxes, and pagers have afforded the opportunity to communicate so easily that you are bombarded with contact. You often confront crowds at the malls, office complexes, and fast food restaurants that you frequent. Within your home, simultaneously played television sets, CD players, and video games can be creating a constant din. The sensory stimulation is unrelenting. You would think that you are a human *doing* rather than a human *being*.

However, when you stop doing and allow yourself to *be* in the moment you afford yourself a rich opportunity for spiritual growth. Solitude provides the forum for this to happen. It is when you remove yourself from the *busy-ness* of daily life that you can be still and quiet enough to truly communicate with God, to pray and speak to Him, and to hear the messages He is communicating to you. Seeking solitude was important for Jesus, who took time from His significant work to communicate with God:

        *…He went up on a mountainside by himself to pray.* Matthew 14:23

        *But Jesus often withdrew to lonely places and prayed.* Luke 5:16

If Jesus made time to seek solitude among His profound activities, can you not find time for solitude in your schedule?

## Purpose

The secular world offers you a generous smorgasbord of blueprints for living your life.  Bookshelves are bulging with "how-to" books that can guide you in planning everything from achieving wealth, to exercising, to achieving eternal youth.  The lecture circuit offers a vast array of charismatic speakers who provide formulas for everything from enjoying perfect relationships to realizing your potential.  Well-intentioned friends and family share their perspectives on the best choices for jobs, neighborhoods, and spouses.  Schools steer students to the "right" schools for the "right" careers.  You will not go wanting for advice regarding planning the direction of your life.

However, life is an adventure of God unfolding His special plan for you.  For a Christian, the key words to consider are *God's plan*.  The plans God has for you may be quite different from the type of plans the secular world promotes.  God is less concerned with you accumulating wealth, marrying a trophy spouse, graduating from an Ivy League school, and landing a high-status position than He is with fulfilling His purpose for you.  The foundation of God's purpose for you is your relationship with Him; from this stems His desire for you to obey, glorify, honor, love, and serve Him.  He then guides you as you walk your unique path in actualizing your purpose.

Living your purpose aligned with God's call may cause you to take actions that are inconsistent with the secular world's views of success.  Consider the following example:

*Frank burst from college with a bright future ahead of him.  His degree in computer programming enabled him to land a job with a major corporation shortly after graduation and the small band that he and some of his friends had formed just for fun had gained ample attention to enable them to earn a substantial income from playing music on weekends.  Frank's impressive corporate position during the week and highly-visible profile in the clubs on weekends attracted gorgeous women and hard-partying friends.  With fame, money, women, and good times, Frank was the envy of his peers.*

*Frank's life was sailing along without a hitch until Beth, a new computer programmer, was hired. Beth had immigrated to the United States from Korea just five years earlier and carried a strong accent.  By comparison to the women in Frank's circles, Beth was not terribly attractive.  Further, Beth was deaf.*

*Within a short time, Frank became fascinated with Beth.  As Frank learned more about this unusual woman, he was touched by challenges she faced in surviving an abusive childhood, completing college, coming to a new country, and living independently.  One day he timidly asked her how she managed to overcome these obstacles.  Without hesitating, Beth responded, "It was Jesus Christ, not I.  He led me every step of the way. All I needed to do was trust, have faith, and love Him."  These words caused something to stir inside of Frank.  He had been raised as a Christian but never understood faith like this.*

*As the months passed, Frank deepened his relationship with Beth and began attending church with her. He was awakened to a new relationship with Jesus, too.  As his prayer life deepened, it became clear to him that he was being stirred in a new direction.*

*Beth and Frank married.  They both continue to work for the same corporation, but in their free time have started a ministry for disabled persons which has become their true passion.  Frank left his band and the kicks associated with their nightclub gigs and now leads a band that uses contemporary music to spread the gospel.  Many of Frank's friends were surprised that of all the beauties he could have chosen, he married a rather plain looking deaf woman and is willing to spend his free time spreading the gospel rather than reaping the money and fame that staying with his former band could have yielded. Yet, Frank is at peace and has never been happier.*

By worldly standards, Frank seems somewhat foolish. He is not capitalizing on his assets and skills to enjoy beautiful women, peak earnings, and an exciting lifestyle. By kingdom standards, however, Frank has aligned his life with God's purpose for him and has discovered deeper and fuller rewards than he ever imagined.

Discovering your purpose begins not by charting a course, but by developing a relationship---with the Lord. It isn't about what you do and achieve, but whom you revere and follow. The realization of your purpose may take different paths at different times in your life, but it needs to be guided by the Lord's will.

## Connection

A right relationship with God is essential for a right relationship with yourself and others. God desires a personal relationship with you. He does not want you to view Him as an untouchable distant power but as a dear loved one. The earliest descriptions of God's interactions with humans reflect His desire for a direct, intimate relationship. For example, the Lord spoke to Moses *as a man speaks to his friend* (Exodus 33:11). He wants to make His abundant love available to you and in turn asks only that you love and obey Him.

Making the space and time in your life for God is essential to your intimate relationship with him. Establishing a daily time to be in prayer and meditation with the Lord, experiencing regular periods of solitude, and studying Scripture are among the ways you can connect more fully with God. (The next chapter will discuss these practices in detail.)

Connection with yourself is an important aspect of health. This entails a realistic appraisal of your sense of worth, motivators, thoughts, and feelings. Characteristics can exist that do not serve you or the Lord well. This conversation between two neighbors exemplifies some of the problems that can exist.

*Mark had just parked his car when he noticed Tom, his next door neighbor, pull in his driveway with a brand new Mercedes Benz. Mark walked over to congratulate Tom on his latest acquisition. "Wow…she is a beauty!" exclaimed Mark. "You bet," replied Tom, "and fully loaded with every imaginable option." "Can't hide money, can you?" teased Mark.*

*"Mark you earn the same as I. "How come you don't treat yourself to a new luxury car instead of buying the economy models?" asked Tom.*

*"Well Tom," Mark responded, "I personally don't think God wants me to use my money to buy fancy things for myself. I just don't deserve it. After all, my old Chevy will take me to the same places as your new Mercedes. I'd rather have a seat in heaven in the future than one in a Mercedes today."*

*"The way I see it," Tom quipped, "God has nothing to do with it. He didn't leave his house at the crack of dawn and put in ten hours a day at a crazy job, I did! I earned it, so who better than I should enjoy it?"*

Tom's perspective that he alone is responsible for receiving and enjoying the material blessings in his life reflects an overestimation of himself.  It runs contrary to Paul's directive to *not think of yourself more highly than you ought, but think of yourself with sober judgment…* (Romans 12:3).  Yet, Mark's attitude leaves much to be desired as well for he is implying that he doesn't deserve to spend the money he has earned, and that God doesn't want people to enjoy nice things.  Neither the extremes of an inflated ego nor a lack of self-worth is desirable.  It is useful to examine yourself to identify misguided attitudes.

Once you are in a right relationship with the Lord and in touch with yourself, you will be in a position to enjoy a healthy connection to others.  You are part of a spiritual family, a kingdom of brothers and sisters:…*so in Christ we who are many form one body, and each member belongs to all the others.* (Romans 12:5).  In comparing the body of believers to the human body, Paul described the relationship and interconnectedness that people have to one another.  The Lord wants you to connect with others and not live in isolation; this would be a form of bondage to yourself and Him---bondage that He does not desire.

Connection with others offers concrete health benefits, also.  The past two decades have shown a growth in our understanding of *psychoneuroimmunology*---a branch of science that describes the relationship of one's psychological state to the immune system.  Studies have found that:

- Social support reduces the negative psychological and physiological effects of stress[2]
- Emotional support from family and friends buffers stressful life events, reduces the risk of depression, and hastens recovery from depression[3]
- People recovering from heart attacks who had emotional support were less likely to die than persons without any source of support[4]
- Women with metastatic breast cancer who participated in a support group where they could share experiences, feelings, and advice lived twice as long as comparable women who did not attend support groups[5]
- Social isolation of primates adversely affects the immune system function and increases susceptibility to disease[6]

Extensive research supports what God has revealed centuries ago:  living in a right relationship to Him, self, and others has multiple benefits.

The next chapter will explore specific ways to incorporate healthy practices into your lifestyle.

## Study Questions

1. How can reliance on medical technology be just as dishonoring to God as engaging in an alternative therapy that calls to spirits in nature to heal?
2. Examine a group in which you are a member (e.g., family, work group, committee). How are the various spiritual gifts represented? What are the risks of not having a good representation of the various spiritual gifts?
3. What are some of the consequences  you witness in society of people violating biblical principles of sexuality?
4. What are some ways that you can use your purpose to fulfill God's purpose?
5. Pay attention to television commercials and advertisements. In what way is the message conveyed that doing is superior to being?

## Related scriptures to pray

Exodus 33:11
Isaiah 58
Hosea 4:6
Psalm 25:12
Proverbs 3:7-8
      17:22
Ecclesiastes 2:24
Matthew 5:27-30
      5:40-42
      6:16-18
      6:24-31
      12:48-50
      16:26
Luke 6:37-38
John 10:10
      14:21
Romans 12:3-5
Acts 13:2
      14:23
      20: 34-38
Ephesians 3:16-19
1 Corinthians 6:20
      12:12-19
Philippians 3:19
1 Timothy 4:1-4
3 John 2

# CHAPTER 5
# ACQUIRE HEALTHY HABITS

In the previous chapters you evaluated your health status and learned about basic practices that promote holistic health.  Now, your challenge is to identify the areas in which you need to make some changes and begin taking actions to do so.  Review the self-assessment that you completed earlier so that you'll be ready to use that information to develop your action plan.

**Rest Well**

Let's begin by looking at your typical day.  Do you awaken refreshed and ready to face the day or with the feeling that you could use several more hours of sleep?  If you find that you lack energy and enthusiasm examine your self-assessment for factors that could be interfering with your sleep and rest, such as:

- high fat, high sugar diet
- insufficient daytime activities
- too many or too lengthy daytime naps
- too much caffeine
- too much alcohol intake
- poorly managed pain
- breathing or circulatory conditions
- urinary tract disorders
- depression
- anxiety
- medications
- dissatisfaction or troubles with your job or relationships
- feeling disconnected from God, spiritually deplete

See if you've checked off any of these items on your assessment and consider the relationship they may have to your sleep and rest pattern.

There are some practical ways you can promote sleep and rest such as:

- establishing a regular bedtime
- meditating on Scripture
- getting some exercise in the late afternoon and early evening
- limiting caffeine and alcohol intake
- spending some time outdoors during the day
- drinking a decaffeinated herbal tea (e.g., chamomile, valerian)
- adjusting the environment (e.g., controlling noise, reducing lighting)
- taking a warm bath about one hour before bedtime
- receiving a massage

If you are having trouble sleeping, you need to explore the reason, so that you can do something about that.

*Over lunch, several friends were discussing how "middle age was catching up with them" because they were turning into bed earlier and earlier each night. With that, Tim pulled a brochure from his pocket. "I just heard about this co-enzyme supplement used for jet lag and chronic fatigue syndrome," Tim shared, "and I'm thinking of using it." "You don't have chronic fatigue syndrome and you haven't been on a plane this year," his friends teasingly responded. "I know," said Tim, "but I haven't slept well for months."*

*Several months prior, Tim's wife returned to work full-time. On closer inspection, Tim's sleep problems could stem from his feelings about shifting family roles and responsibilities, his wife's reduced availability, or other issues pertaining to his wife's job.*

Tim could benefit more from praying for clarity and exploring the underlying issue than treating the symptoms.


## Build in Prayer

A wonderful routine to establish is to spend some time with the Lord before launching into your daily routines. I find that as an early-riser, my best time for prayer is in the early morning hours before my husband stirs, the phone begins ringing, and the responsibilities of the day get going. Spending this quiet time with the Lord starts my day on a grounded, peaceful footing and enables me to be more aware of His presence with me throughout the day than if I rushed into my daily activities without prayer. I compare it to having a guest in my home who will be accompanying me throughout the day. With this special person by my side, I tend to be more thoughtful of my words and actions than when I'm alone. Likewise, a conscious effort to connect with the Lord in the morning and invite Him to accompany me through the day cause me to be aware of the way in which my words and actions affect Him.

It is helpful to schedule time for prayer in the same manner as any other important or essential activity in your life. If you think you'll have trouble squeezing prayer time into your morning, ask the Lord to assist you. The time you spend with the Lord can help you to get focused and centered, and approach the day with a positive attitude, knowing you will not have to face your challenges alone.

Incorporate prayer into your day as much as possible. On your way to a meeting or to work, ask the Lord for guidance, patience, and understanding. As you're sitting in rush hour traffic going nowhere fast, use the time to offer prayers. Communicate with the Lord as you take a walk. Affirm your love for God throughout the day. Confess your wrongdoings and keep a short account with God.

There is no right or wrong way to pray. God is more interested in your honest, open relationship with Him than he is in you following a specific protocol for praying. There are as many various styles of prayer as there are people who pray. Prayer can include talking (aloud or silently), meditating on scripture verses, listening for God to speak, crying, chanting, singing, or being acutely aware of the present moment. Its components can include acknowledgement of the wonders of God's power, grace, and mercy; expressions of adoration and appreciation for all God has offered; petitions to God for specific needs and guidance; confession of sins; and requests on behalf of others. Regardless of the style or content of your prayers, make them a frequent and active part of your daily routines.

## Eat Wisely

In the previous chapter the components of a nutritious diet were reviewed. The challenge is to establish eating habits that support the principles of good nutrition. A basic step is to allow yourself time to eat regular, nutritious meals. There is a risk that if you skip a meal you'll go for the candy bar or chips when you begin to feel hunger pangs, so schedule meals. A review of your typical food intake on your self-assessment can help you to spot bad habits.

Breakfast is important. You don't need to consume a large breakfast, just a smart one. Rather than coffee and a sweet bun, eat some fresh fruit, grain cereal with skim milk or yogurt, and juice. After breakfast you may want to take a good multivitamin supplement. Although the statement is made that "if you eat right you don't need a supplement", the reality is that most of us do not eat right. It can be quite challenging to consume the proper quantity and quality of food to obtain the recommended daily allowance of most nutrients. Few of us have the benefit of eating freshly picked fruits and vegetables; the longer the period between when these items were picked and when they reach your table, the greater the loss of nutrients. Further, the processing and cooking of food causes some vitamins and minerals to be lost. A daily multivitamin supplement can compensate for these factors and assure you get the basic micronutrients that you need.

Although a single daily multivitamin supplement can be beneficial, don't overdo a good thing. *Megavitamin therapy*---also called orthomolecular therapy---has become popular. This involves taking high doses of vitamins, minerals, and amino acids. There are claims that megavitamin therapy can help a wide range of health conditions, such as attention deficit disorder, schizophrenia, and allergies, however, research is inconclusive at this time. In addition to ingesting costly supplements that you don't need, using high doses of vitamins and minerals can be dangerous. For example, large doses of vitamin E can thin the blood and cause bleeding; excess vitamin D can increase the blood pressure and cause muscle and bone pain; high intakes of vitamin A can cause anemia and joint pain. Avoid megavitamin therapy unless you are under the direction of a health care professional.

Be sure to buy your supplements from reputable sources and to check the expiration dates. Read the labels carefully as one manufacturer's product may require 3 tablets to consume the same dose that you could obtain from one tablet of another product---which can be a considerable factor in cost! Unfortunately, the quality of supplements can vary from distributor to distributor, and a higher cost doesn't assure a higher quality. If you seriously want to research the quality of supplements produced by various companies you may want to visit the website of ConsumerLab.com, a company that conducts independent product reviews. (General information is free; a nominal fee is charged to be a subscriber and have access to a wider range of information and services.)

In addition to the *what* of your eating habits, also consider the *how*. Do you gulp food down without giving your taste buds a chance to detect what is passing through? Are you mindlessly shoving food in your mouth while you're plastered in front of the television set? Have you created your version of Meals on Wheels by hastily eating while negotiating rush hour traffic with a carload of kids? Enjoying the dining *experience* is an important aspect of eating wisely. You needn't set the table with your finest china, and serve elaborate meals every day to enjoy the dining experience, but little niceties can make a difference. My husband and I are friends with a wonderful couple who demonstrate this point. They work full time and have busy schedules, yet they've committed that barring unusual circumstances, their dinners at home will be by candlelight. They may be eating leftovers or carryout foods, but they do it by candlelight with the lights dimmed. This relatively minor touch creates an atmosphere that allows them to transition from their busy-ness to calmness. I wonder how many ordinary mealtimes could become dining experiences with minor environmental modifications like candles or soft music.

Eating also can become a dining experience by taking the time to enjoy what you're eating. Try experimenting for a day in making a conscious effort to identify all the sensations of all the food you eat: the crunching sound as you bite into an apple, the aroma of coffee, the smooth surface of a tomato, the ridges of a raisin as you roll in on your tongue, the different flavors and colors of the food you encounter in one meal. God certainly could have made a single food substance to fulfill our nutritional needs, however, He chose to bless us with a wide range of flavors, colors, textures, scents, and even sounds to stimulate our senses and offer greater pleasure to us as we ate. To take the time to enjoy food is one way to show appreciation to God for this blessing---and to derive greater health benefits from eating.

*Weight Control*

According to the National Institutes of Health more than 2/3 of adults and 1/3 of children and adolescents are overweight. About 1/3 of overweight adults are considered obese (having a body mass index equal to or greater than 30).; 1 in 20 adults is extremely obese. Although genetic factors, some medications (e.g., steroids, tricyclic antidepressants, antihypertensives), and a few diseases can cause some people to become obese, most people develop this problem because their caloric input exceeds their caloric expenditure. A sedentary lifestyle and high-fat, high-carbohydrate diet are significant risk factors for obesity.

Even in the absence of genetic factors, disease, and drug effects, some people have been obese for most of their lives. This frequently is related to the role of food and eating in their families. My own background exemplifies this.  I am from a Greek family and was raised in a Greek community.  If you've ever known Greeks or visited Greece, you probably understand that the Greeks have some fantastic foods and they love to eat.  In my childhood home, my stay-at-home mom prepared fine meals just about every day.  (In fact, I can remember as a kid begging my mother to please stop serving us mousaka, pasticcio, souvlaki, and all that other "awful Greek stuff" and give us some all-American hot dogs, burgers, and canned spaghetti.)  You can believe that after spending hours preparing those wonderful dishes, my mother wanted to see the fruits of her labor consumed, so there was considerable pressure put on my brother and me to eat.  Neither he nor I had particularly large appetites (thankfully!) so dinner table battles were frequent as our parents urged us to eat and we resisted.  To make matters worse, every social encounter involved food---and not just light snacks but a fully loaded table with Greek meatballs, feta cheese, loaves of crusty bread, olives, baklava, and on and on and on.  To enter a Greek home and not sample the food that was offered was considered a major insult.  When most of your family and social acquaintances are Greek this means life nearly becomes a moveable feast.  A reasonable appetite and high energy level enabled me to escape becoming obese; however, I have relatives and friends who were less fortunate and are living with the consequences.

The beliefs and practices you developed about eating from your family also may have been built on erroneous information.  My husband describes an ongoing battle at his childhood dinner table---where potatoes were served daily---between his father and brother.  His brother wanted to eat generous portions of green vegetables and skip the potatoes.  His dad believed you needed the heartiness of potatoes rather than "those green vegetables that wouldn't do you any good or put meat on your bones", and scolded the boy for not consuming his daily pile of the starchy vegetable.  Be it the misinformation gained about the nutritional value of certain foods, unhealthy cooking methods, or unsound eating habits, the foundation our families laid strongly influence our lifelong eating habits and can be a significant factor in obesity.

Another contributing factor to obesity is that food may be meeting other needs in your life.  For example, you may lack purpose, love, or relationships in your life and fulfill these emotional needs by seeking the comfort of food (and usually not the carrots and celery variety!).  I once led a weight control group for women in a community health program.  Many of these women were middle-aged homemakers who no longer had children at home and who shared little interests with their husbands.  They spent many hours alone in their homes while their husbands were gone, working, bowling, and socializing with the guys at the local tavern.  For the most part, they passed their time watching television, snacking as they did.  Thus began the unfortunate cycle:

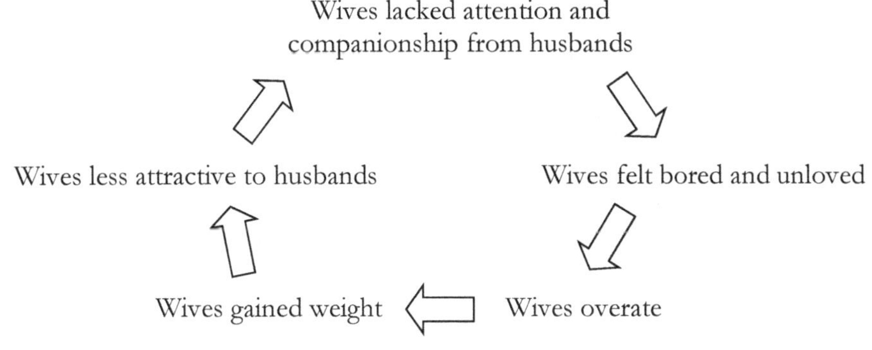

Food was used by these women to numb the pain of unsatisfying marriages and boredom. Although education and guidance in dietary modifications were offered to this group, the more significant ways that I impacted their weight loss were to guide them in exploring their emotional reasons for eating, encourage them to become involved in activities outside the home, and help them learn ways to express their needs and communicate more effectively with their husbands.

In that same weight control group another issue arose which can influence the ability to lose weight: lack of family support for the goal of weight loss. There was a woman in the group whose situation reflected this. Irma, who barely stood five feet tall, weighed 225 pounds. She shared that she had weighed about 110 pounds when she had married 19 years ago and progressively gained weight until she reached her current level of obesity. Irma's beautiful features made it easy to imagine that she must have turned quite a few heads back then. Initially, Irma was showing a weight loss at her weekly weigh-ins but about six weeks into the program, she hit a plateau and then began gaining weight again. At first, Irma pretended to have no idea why this was happening, but then confessed that she had been "slipping". In exploring this with Irma, I learned that just when people started to notice that she was losing her weight, her husband began bringing home fattening goodies on a daily basis. The longstanding problem of weak willpower compounded by strong urging by her husband to "go ahead and have some; I bought this just for you!" caused her to succumb to temptation. With the group's support, Irma armed herself to try to get on track and asked her husband to avoid bringing home any edible treats. Although her husband ignored her request, the group's support helped her to follow her diet and she again began to shed the pounds. I then received a telephone call from Irma informing me that her husband was making her drop out of the group. "He told me he likes me just the way I am and that I don't have to lose any weight." Further into the conversation Irma revealed that her husband had hinted that if she got thin, she may no longer be satisfied with him or may want to return to work rather than be at home for him. His insecurities caused him to sabotage her diet efforts. Obviously, the understanding and support of one's family are key ingredients to successfully changing eating habits.

If obesity is an issue with you, reflect on your beliefs about food, cultural influences, family dynamics, relationships, and emotional needs that influence your overeating. Ask the Lord to give you insights and direction. List the factors you've identified and write some realistic steps you can take to change them. You may find it beneficial to recruit a friend to assist you with this process. Before starting to diet, get a complete physical examination. In addition to learning about any special precautions you need to heed while dieting based on your unique health status, an examination can unveil health conditions that are contributing to your weight gain, such as endocrine disturbances or a tumor.

Avoid extreme diets or weight loss fads as these are difficult to sustain on a long-term basis and could pose serious health risks. The goal is not to take off as much weight as possible as quickly as you can, but to make lifestyle modifications that can help to improve your overall health and maintain your weight within a healthy range. Some principles to guide you are offered in Table 7.

An important aspect to remember if you struggle with obesity is that God loves you regardless of your body size. And, He offers hope and support to you in your efforts to gain the self-discipline to resist making food your god.

---

**Table 7**
**Tips for Weight Reduction**

- Consult with your health care practitioner to determine if there are any factors you must consider as you begin a weight reduction program.
- Review your beliefs, attitudes, and experiences that contribute to unhealthy eating habits. Reflect on the reasons you overeat. Ask the Lord to reveal specific issues to you.
- Elicit your family's support.
- Keep a food diary for several days prior to starting your diet. Examine it for factors that contribute to obesity, such as skipping a meal and then binging on sweets, consuming a disproportionate amount of fats.
- Determine your desired calorie intake and plot how this will be divided over the day.
- Follow a sensible eating plan. Avoid starvation diets, fads, or over-the-counter drugs for weight loss.
- Consume a balanced diet that includes at least 100 gram of carbohydrates and 50 to 100 grams of protein (predominately from foods that are low in saturated fat and cholesterol).
- Take a daily multivitamin supplement.
- Avoid high-protein diets. Although they can cause initial weight loss and reduce appetite because the high fat content satisfies you, high protein diets can increase your risk for cardiovascular disease, osteoporosis, and perhaps cancer. The extra excretion of body fluids caused by these diets also increases the workload of your kidneys.
- Consume foods with a low *glycemic index*. The glycemic index ranks foods by how they affect blood sugar. Foods with a low glycemic index break down slowly, and consequently, release their energy at a slower rate which in turn, helps you feel fuller longer. These foods also help to keep the blood sugar stable which prevents you from feeling hungry. Foods with a low glycemic index include foods such as whole grain breads, pumpernickel, all bran cereal, toasted muesli, yogurt, milk, apples, oranges, peaches, lentils, soybeans, and baked beans.
- Begin each day with a prayer for strength and discipline to adhere to your dietary plan.
- Start or increase your current exercise program to increase your metabolic rate. In addition, take advantage of opportunities in your daily routine to boost your activity level (e.g., walking stairs instead of taking an elevator, parking at the farthest space on the lot).
- Drink at least 8 glasses of water throughout the day. If it is difficult for you to drink that much plain water, try drinking flavored seltzer water or decaffeinated herbal teas. (A cup of peppermint tea taken before meals can help in reducing appetite.
- Keep plenty of celery and carrots on hand to munch on between meals.
- If you slip off your diet, don't be too hard on yourself. Changing any habit is difficult. Explore the reasons for straying from your plan and try to address them, including specifically praying for strength to avoid having them interfere with your goal again.
- Rejoice in your progress.

---

## Fast

The chemicals that are consumed in the average American diet cause toxins to accumulate in the body that can lead to a variety of ill effects.  One method to eliminate these toxins is by fasting.  Fasting has been used since the earliest of times to cleanse the body and sharpen the spirit.  The Bible shows that more than 800 years before the birth of Jesus Christ, Jesoshaphat called upon the people of Judah to fast so that they could seriously focus on their sin and pray for God's help (2 Chronicles 20:3-4).  When returning to Jerusalem, Ezra and his co-travelers fasted and prayed to seek the spiritual preparation for their journey (Ezra 8:23).  Jesus fasted for 40 days and nights in the desert (Matthew 4:2) and emphasized the right reasons to fast:  to spend time in prayer and reflect on God's blessings (Matthew 6:16-18).  Jesus urged those who fasted to *"not look somber"* or *"disfigure their faces to show men they are fasting"* but to look and act as normally as possible.  This remains solid advice to follow in your fasting.  By going about business as usual and not drawing attention to your fast, you will be less likely to be preoccupied with symptoms and can ease your burden.  Fasting teaches self-discipline and offers the opportunity to turn your thoughts to God.  (If you do nothing more than use the time you would have spent in purchasing, preparing, and eating food in prayer you have done well!)

There are various types of fasts that you can do ranging from the ingestion of nothing but water, to consuming only juices and fruits.  Fasting can last anywhere from one day to several weeks.  If you are healthy and there is no medical problem that would be affected by fasting, you should experience no difficulty with a two-day fast consisting of only water intake or a five-day fast in which only water and juices are ingested.  Prolonged fasts or fasts in the presence of health conditions need to be conducted under the supervision of a health professional.  Fasting usually is not advised for persons with diabetes, hypoglycemia, eating disorders, malnutrition, cancer, infectious diseases, renal or liver disease, ulcerative colitis, or bronchial asthma; women who are pregnant should not fast.

Fasting stimulates a cleansing and removal of toxins from the body which can cause some physical effects, including:

- coated tongue
- unpleasant taste
- halitosis
- increased body odor
- skin dryness
- headache
- fatigue
- dizziness
- insomnia
- nausea
- aching joints
- flu-like symptoms
- reduced pulse and blood pressure.

In some persons, an irregular heartbeat can occur.  A several pound weight loss is common.

You don't need to drastically modify your activities for short-term fasts, although it is best to avoid strenuous exercise.  You may want to schedule extra rest periods on the days when you fast.  A good fluid intake during the fast is essential.

Good personal hygiene is important while fasting.  As toxins are eliminated through the skin, frequent bathing is useful, including gently scrubbing of the skin with a soft brush.  Frequent oral hygiene is needed, as well.  (Rinsing the mouth with lemon juice can reduce tongue coating and unpleasant tastes.  Be sure to follow this with a rinse with water to protect your teeth's enamel from the acidic effects of the lemon juice.)

There is some belief that the elimination of toxins and other beneficial effects of fasting can be accomplished in a gentler way with a *cleansing diet* such as:
Breakfast:  low-sugar fruit eaten whole
One hour before lunch:  water
Lunch:  steamed vegetables and a grain product
One hour before supper:  fresh vegetable juice
Supper:  noncream soup or salad
This low-fat, high-fiber vegetarian diet provides a continuous cleansing effect without the stress of a fast.

Fasting is a spiritual discipline, therefore spiritual preparation accompanies physical preparation for a fast.  Prior to fasting. pray for God's guidance for the type of fast you need.  Ask God to help you identify your sins so that you can use your fast as a time to confess and pray for repentance.  While fasting, think about the attributes of God and the ways in which He has blessed your life.  Be open to the voice of the Holy Spirit.  Expect spiritual opposition as your bodily symptoms challenge you to forfeit your fast; pray for God's help as you resist the temptation to prematurely break your fast.  Discipline your mind to focus on your desire for spiritual growth rather than your sacrifice of food, remembering that: *Blessed are those who hunger and thirst for righteousness for they will be filled* (Matthew 5:6).

## Exercise

Consider the amount of exercise you get in a typical day.  If you're not doing so at present, try to schedule some regular form of exercise (e.g., walking, playing ball, an aerobics class) at least several times during the week---or, ideally, daily.  If you're unaccustomed to exercising start with a 20 minutes session and then progress to 45 minutes as your tolerance and condition improve.  In addition, take advantage of opportunities to increase your exercise during your routine day; this could include:
- walking the stairs instead of taking the elevator
- parking in the farthest spot from the building
- using part of your lunch time to take a short walk
- taking a few minutes each hour to stretch and bend

When doing exercises for cardiopulmonary endurance---such as jogging, walking, cycling, swimming, and other forms of aerobic exercises---it is beneficial to determine your *heart rate during exercise* to assure that the rate stays within a safe range.  To do this, subtract your age from the figure 220 to obtain your *maximum heart rate* and multiply that answer by 70% to obtain your *target heart rate..*  Your heart rate should stay in a range of 10 beats of your target heart rate during exercise. For example, if you are 45 years of age, your heart rate should fall within 112 and 133 beats per minute based on the following calculation:

$$
\begin{array}{rl}
220 & \\
-\ \ 45 & \\
\hline
175 & \textit{Maximum heart rate} \\
\times\ \ 0.7 & \\
\hline
122.5 & \textit{Target heart rate}
\end{array}
$$

If your heart rate during exercise is more than 10 beats above the target heart rate the exercise should be reduced the next time it is done.  If your heart rate is more than 10 beats lower than the target heart rate, you should increase the intensity of your exercise the next time to assure you are obtaining the best cardiopulmonary benefit.  (Heart rate monitors can be used as alternatives to manually taking your pulse.)  Try to gradually increase the intensity of your exercise.  You're on safe ground as long as you are able to carry on a conversation without experiencing symptoms of overexertion (e.g., chest pain, severe shortness of breath, dizziness, nausea).

It is important for you to develop an exercise plan that you can sustain long-term.  This must be taken into account when you are considering joining a gym, committing to a class, or laying out a large sum of money for equipment.  Here's an example that worked for one mom of young children:

> *Debbie is a mother of two children under the age of 3. Last year she enrolled in an aerobics class on Wednesday evenings but found that on most Wednesday evenings either her husband worked overtime or a child was sick, limiting her attendance.  She purchased exercise videos but just couldn't get motivated to use them.  When discussing this problem with other young moms in the neighborhood, she discovered she wasn't alone in facing obstacles to exercise.  When she suggested that the moms commit to meeting Monday, Wednesday, and Friday mornings for a half hour exercise time the other moms responded enthusiastically.  The women take turns leading exercises which have varied from following a video to taking a brisk walk with the children in strollers to doing aerobics with worship music as a background.  Each mom takes a turn at being the "on-call mother" to attend to any needs of the children that surface during the exercise time so that the other moms can have an uninterrupted period.  The peer support has helped Debbie stick with her exercise program and has provided wonderful fellowship.*

## Manage Stress

Develop effective ways to manage the stress which you're certain to experience in an average day.  Getting proper rest and eating a nutritious diet can boost your ability to manage stress, as can doing deep breathing exercises, slowly counting to ten, diverting your attention, scheduling your time realistically, and saying a short prayer.  Some of the items listed under *Emotional and Spiritual* on your self-assessment can be the cause and the result of stress, so see if you have any of them listed and try to examine how you can improve them.

*Solitude*

Carving out time alone is a wonderful way to keep stress from overwhelming your life. Although the spiritual discipline of solitude is not intended to be a stress management technique, solitary time can help you to clear your head, gain insight into your life and your relationships, and deepen your relationship to Jesus. During periods of silence you can gain insights into behaviors that keep your life from being balanced and fruitful. You can seek solitude in several ways:

- Schedule a day of complete solitude once each month. Go away if you can; if that is not possible, stay home and leave the kids with a friend, unplug the phone, refrain from checking email or regular mail. (Before claiming that you just couldn't find a day each month to be alone, just consider the time you spend in unessential activities, such as window shopping and watching television, and try to shift your priorities.)
- Build at least one-half hour of personal quiet time into each day. The morning, before the rest of the family rises, can be a good time and has the added advantage of getting you centered to face the day.
- If you work or are engaged in activities outside the home, decompress and take 15 minutes alone between the time you come home and the time you start home chores.
- Designate a room or chair that the rest of your family can identify as your "quiet time place." When you occupy this space it signifies that this is your time alone and that you shouldn't be interrupted.
- Reduce routine distractions. Turn off the car radio and use driving time for reflection. Avoid having television and music playing as background noise.

By making time and space available for you and God to interact, you invite opportunities for Him to work in your life.

## Enjoy Work

Work plays such a major role in the lives of most people that the relationship between your work and your health warrants examination. Do you view your work as purposeful, satisfying, and energizing, or does it drain your body, mind, and spirit? One difficulty you could face if your work is more burdensome than rewarding is that your work isn't suited for your giftedness.

At our birth, the Holy Spirit gave each of us different types of *spiritual gifts* (Table 8). No one gift is more important than another. All are needed in the kingdom of Christ. However, you can feel out of balance if you are placed in roles in which you lack opportunities to exercise your gift or where you're expected to show strength in an area in which you are not gifted. Pastor Andy's experience is an example:

> *While attending a church service with family in a neighboring state, an elder from a young church heard a pastor deliver one of the most powerful sermons he had heard in a long time. The pastor, Andy Alson, was a mild-mannered, unassuming man in a crowd, but on the altar he let loose with a dynamic teaching style that was evidently empowered by the Holy Spirit. Knowing his church desperately needed this type of leadership, the elder didn't hesitate to contact the other elders of his home church and tell them of his find. After several visits and exploratory meetings, Andy was offered the position of senior pastor. He and his family saw this as a positive, logical next move.*
> *At the new church, Andy shared teaching responsibilities with two other pastors, and in addition, was administratively responsible for all operations. The congregation was moved by his*

*teaching and appreciated his "approachable" style.*

*In a short time, the few hundred church members grew to a few thousand. The six person staff that was present when Andy came to the church had grown to thirty-five, representing a wide range of functions and ministries. As the people and activities grew, so did the problems: inter-ministry conflict, employees who were functioning below par, varying opinions on how to manage the growing body. Andy's nonconfrontational style and lack of ease with managerial functions prevented him from exercising the strong leadership that the church---as a complex organization now---needed. His teaching was more powerful than ever, but his administrative deficits were causing havoc operationally. Further, Andy was feeling increasingly frustrated at being burdened with tasks that he didn't feel comfortable doing and began questioning if he should consider finding a position in another church.*

*It took an outside consultant to shed light on one of the major problems: Andy's gifts were teaching and evangelism, not administration. In fact, no one on the leadership staff had a gift of administration. Realizing this deficit, the church hired a lay administrator to direct its operations and freed Andy to focus on teaching. Within a short time church operations were being well-managed and Andy felt a new level of excitement, evidenced by an even more dynamic teaching style than he had shared previously.*

Having a poor fit between your giftedness and your work can lead you to be frustrated and ineffective. Granted, you may not be able to find the ideal job for your giftedness. For example, you may have the gift of teaching and find delight being in a classroom setting yet find that a teacher's salary is insufficient to support your family's expenses. If your family has determined that it can do nothing more to reduce expenses and you need to be employed at a job that produces higher earnings, perhaps you can seek a position in a corporation's human resources department where your gift can be used; another option is to teach Sunday school or lead a Bible study at your church so that you have an outlet for expression of your gift.

---

## Table 8  Spiritual Gifts

Wisdom
Knowledge
Teaching
Administration
Leading
Helping
Mercy
Faith
Healing
Prophecy
Evangelism

---

## Connect with Nature

The first chapter of Genesis describes how God took nothingness and created light, sky, sun, moon, stars, water, plants, trees, fish, birds, and a wide array of living creatures.  Our Almighty Father took pride in His creation, judging it to be good.  He then gave the apex of His creation, man and woman, the gift of this vast, wondrous creation---to inhabit, tend, and enjoy.

It is useful for your physical, mental, and spiritual well-being to spend time enjoying nature each day. This could be accomplished through a walk in the park, driving home from work on a scenic route (even if it takes a little longer!), gardening, or sitting outside on your porch.  Take a few minutes to allow your senses to experience the wonderful surroundings:   listen to birds chirping, take in a deep breath and notice the scent of the grass and flowers, stroke the petal of a flower.

Connection with nature fosters your connection to God, also.  It is difficult to see the spectacular colors of a sunset, gaze across a body of water that seems to go on forever, hear birds chirping their unique songs, or smell the fragrance of blossoming flowers without feeling awestruck at the superb craftsmanship of God. You honor Him by enjoying the products of His creation.

## Laugh!

*A cheerful heart is good medicine, but a crushed spirit dries up the bones.*  Proverbs 17:22

Humor and optimism have a positive impact on your health state.  The act of laughing produces physiological effects that can be beneficial; these effects include:

- Increased heart rate and circulation
- Increased respirations and oxygenation of tissues
- Exercise of thoracic and abdominal muscles
- Release of endorphins which is helpful in improving mood, reducing pain sensations, decreasing anxiety, and relieving muscle tension
- Increased metabolism
- Stimulation of the immune system

Find ways for laughter to permeate your life and the lives you touch. Share jokes and funny stories. If you're not skilled at remembering or delivering jokes, try keeping a scrapbook of clippings of funny stories and jokes that you can tap when needed. Include an abundance of comedies among your movie selections. Rent videos of old *I Love Lucy, Candid Camera, Marx Brothers, Laurel and Hardy,* and other classics, as well as more contemporary sitcoms. Read humorous books. Spend time with children. Be playful and smile often.

Very importantly, don't take yourself too seriously. Be willing to laugh at yourself, particularly when you make stupid mistakes. You have a choice as to the manner in which you react to the unpleasant incidents in your life. You can become angry and complain, or find the humor in the situation and take it lightly. Finding the humor in the situation gives you a sense of control. Further, it influences the mood of those around you and can aid in reducing the stress of yourself and others.

**Be Proactive**

Good health practices also include smart management of your symptoms and illnesses. Review your self-assessment and evaluate some of the conditions and symptoms you've checked. How many of them can you prevent or improve by lifestyle changes, such as changing your diet, increasing your exercise, reducing your intake of alcohol, or managing your stress more effectively? You need to consider some of the reasons that you may not have taken these actions in the past (e.g., lack of knowledge regarding good nutritional practices, poor motivation, family pressures, cultural factors) and try to work on them as you can.

We have become a society that looks for quick and easy relief in a pill. Not all medications are bad; in fact, many drugs have not only enabled people to add years to their lives, but also increase the quality of life to their years. God has revealed these treatments to us to assist in our healing. Yet, there are risks with drugs, serious risks. The side effects of a drug can cause more discomfort than the symptoms for which it was originally prescribed. And, medications can be fatal. These comments are not meant to suggest that you not use medications, but that you use them only when necessary and appropriately. Medications should not be used as a substitute for you taking an active role in your own healing. Reducing junk foods could eliminate your need for antacids; exercising and reducing weight could cause your joints to be less painful and reduce the need for a pain reliever; spending quiet time with the Lord can relieve anxieties and eliminate the need for tranquilizers and sedatives. Some ways to enhance your safety in using drugs are described in Table 9.

---

**Table 9**
**Using Drugs Safely**

- *Try to address the cause of the symptom rather than just treat the symptom.* For example, if you experience indigestion every time you eat fried chicken and find yourself using an antacid to relieve the discomfort, your wisest action is to omit fried chicken from your diet
- *Use measures other than drugs to treat your symptoms when possible.* Instead of using a tranquilizer when feeling stressed, try meditation, a massage, or deep breathing exercises. If you are having a rise in blood pressure, try changing your diet, practicing yoga stretches, and doing progressive relaxation exercises before starting on an antihypertensive drug.
- *Check for potential interactions.* Inform your health care provider of all the prescription and over-the-counter medications you are using before a new drug is prescribed. Review your medications with your pharmacist and ask about potential interactions. If your are taking any medications on a regular basis, do not begin taking a new drug without consulting with your health care provider.
- *Don't self-medicate or use other people's medications.* It is tempting to use your spouse's unfinished antibiotic prescription when you believe you are experiencing the same ailment or to use the remainder of your antibiotics that have been sitting in the medicine cabinet for over one year, but do yourself a favor and don't do it! Dosage requirements can vary from person to person, as well as from year to year in the same person. Also, drug potency changes as a medication sits. Flush unused prescriptions down the toilet.
- *Follow the instructions carefully.* Don't think that if one works two will work better; in some situations, one can work and two can cause serious adverse reactions.
- *Be knowledgeable of the drugs you are using.* For every drug you use, become familiar with the:
  expected actions
  dosage
  schedule and route of administration
  side effects
  adverse reactions
  interactions
  precautions
  special instructions

It could be beneficial for you to keep a written record that contains these facts that you can carry in your wallet or purse. This could prove useful in the event of a medical emergency or when you consult health care professionals.

---

Table 10 offers a few hints to help you acquire healthy patterns. Changing your health habits isn't easy…change seldom is! However, we can't forget that as Christians, we have a duty to care for the bodies, minds, and spirits with which we have been blessed.

*Do you not know that the body is a temple of the Holy spirit, who is in you, whom you have received from God? You were bought at a price. Therefore, honor God with your body.*
1 Corinthians 6: 19-20

---

**Table 10**
**Hints to Aid You in Acquiring Healthy Habits**

- Elicit God's help by praying for strength, patience, and perseverance to improve your health
- Believe that you are able to change and improve your health
- Ask a friend or family member to serve as your coach so that you can have a buddy to offer support and hold you accountable
- Form mental images of the end result you want to achieve (e.g., a thinner body, a more relaxed state)
- Network with others who may be confronting similar challenges to share tips and offer support
- Keep a journal so that you can identify your progress, patterns, and pitfalls
- Use affirmations that describe the goals you will achieve ("I am able to eat a well-balanced diet, I am able to walk for 15 minutes every evening")
- Identify your accomplishments, reward yourself, and praise God
- Pray, pray, pray!

---

## Study Questions

1.  How can many unhealthy practices (e.g., eating poorly, cheating on sleep requirements) be traced to violations of God's will for His people?
2.  What are the differences between loneliness and being alone?
3.  What are some ways that you can celebrate nature?
4.  God has revealed insights into ways that people can heal their bodies from disease (e.g., pharmacological and technological interventions).  How can these treatments be misused in such a way that they are dishonoring to God?

## Related scriptures to pray

Genesis 1
Psalm 19:1-6
      23
      24:1-6
Proverbs 31:10-31
Ecclesiastes 1:1-14
Matthew 6:25-34
      7:7-11
      9:1-8
      14:35-36
Luke 11:1-9

# CHAPTER 6
# NURTURE YOURSELF

When you think of the word nurture you may associate it with investing in your children so they realize their potential or nourishing a garden so it is abundant with flowers and fruits. The nurturing efforts put into young lives and gardens are proactive actions to yield positive results.

*Self-nurturing* is an essential part of a healthy, balanced life. Christ-centered self-nurturing encompasses more than caring for your body, mind, and spirit for the sake of promoting optimal health, function, and well-being. Instead, by taking intentional steps to nurture yourself, you can achieve a closer relationship with God so that He can transform and fully use your life.

## Spiritual Disciplines

The spiritual disciplines provide a solid framework for self-nurturing. Spiritual disciplines are activities in which you intentionally engage that enliven and deepen your relationship to God and His kingdom. Important aspects to understand are that they are *intentional*, that is, done purposefully rather than by chance, and are *focused on the Lord*. An abundant, balanced life demands interaction with a living, personal God that is intentional rather than haphazard. Regular practice of the spiritual disciplines helps you to tap into God's power and be prepared to serve Him. Spiritual disciplines enable you to deepen your understanding and relationship to yourself, as well, to help you to unpeel layers of your composition and understand your core. The result is an achievement of a more abundant life---a deeper life in the spirit.

There are a variety of activities that are regarded as spiritual disciplines. Richard Foster[7] identifies the spiritual disciplines as:

*Inward Disciplines*: meditation, prayer, fasting, study
*Outward Disciplines:* simplicity, solitude, submission, service
*Corporate Disciplines:* confession, worship, guidance, celebration

Dallas Willard[8] took a different approach to categorizing the spiritual disciplines by dividing them into disciplines that disengage us from those life activities that interfere with our relationship with God (Disciplines of Abstinence) and disciplines that immerse us more deeply in God's kingdom (Disciplines of Engagement); his lists include:

> *Disciplines of Abstinence:* solitude, silence, fasting, frugality, chastity, secrecy, sacrifice, watching

> *Disciplines of Engagement:* study, worship, celebration, service, prayer, fellowship, confession, submission

There is nothing mysterious about the practice of spiritual disciplines. The Bible offers fine examples of how Jesus and His disciples wove these practices into their routine lives and instructed others to do so as part of the Christian life. For example:

> After He had dismissed them, He went up on a mountainside by Himself to pray. *Matthew 14:23*

> Going a little farther, He fell to the ground and prayed… *Mark 14:35*

> Therefore, confess your sins to each other and pray for each other so that you may be healed. *James 5:16*

> Let us not give up meeting together… *Hebrews 10:25*

> When He had said this, he knelt down with all of them and prayed… *Acts 21:36*

> Jesus stopped and called them, "What do you want me to do for you?" He asked. *Matthew 21:32*

> …and whoever wants to be first must be your slave---just as the Son of Man did not come to be served, but to serve… *Matthew 20:27*

> But Jesus often withdrew to lonely places and prayed. *Luke 5:16*

Great musicians didn't first pick up their instruments and begin playing in a symphony orchestra. World series baseball players didn't progress from Little League to Major League overnight. Skilled cardiac surgeons didn't take scalpels to people's chests on their first day in medical school. The ease and expertise demonstrated by individuals who have achieved greatness in their fields have come from considerable focus, study, and practice. The behaviors that now seem to come easily and naturally to these talented persons are the result of a considerable investment of time and effort. They ate, slept, and breathed the talent they desired to master. Likewise, your regular focus, study, and practice of the spiritual disciplines can lead you to an abundant life in the kingdom of Christ because you learn that submitting to His will begins to naturally permeate every breathing moment of your existence.

## Prayer

Of all the spiritual disciplines, prayer is the one that probably is most commonly practiced by believers. This communication with the Lord enlivens our faith and nurtures our souls. Although discussed in an earlier chapter, prayer warrants some further attention here.

As simple as it seems, prayer risks being misunderstood.  I recall one of my early experiences in learning to pray---or at least that is what it was labeled.  I was somewhere in the neighborhood of 12 years of age and attending a Greek Orthodox church.  At that time, the full service was spoken in Greek; unfortunately, I neither spoke nor understood Greek.  However, my Sunday school assignment was to learn the Apostle's Creed——in Greek!  My anxiety brewed.  How was I ever going to do this?  I imagined the embarrassment at being the only one among my peers---all of whom were quite fluent in Greek by the way---to  be unable to recite the words.  My Sunday school teacher, sensitive to my plight, volunteered to tutor me in the task.  For several weeks, nearly every other evening, this dedicated woman taught me verse after verse, phonetically.  I'd practice in front of my parents, in front of the mirror, in front of my dog, in front of anything that would stay still long enough to hear me recite in a foreign tongue.  When the time came for me to stand before my class and recite the Creed, I was able to do so.  In fact, I was so impressive that I was selected to recite the Apostle's Creed at the assembly for parents.  My head grew from the compliments I received in my delivery of this prayer.  It wasn't until I reached adulthood that I actually read the Creed in English and understood what I had been saying.

My parroting of foreign words could hardly be considered praying.  Yet, reciting prayers by rote is no more effective a means of prayer either, despite the fact that it is done in one's own language.  Prayer isn't about spurting out impressive sounding scripture but *communicating with God.*  There are many fine books that offer guidance on the process of prayer; however, the basic instructions have been provided by the greatest teacher of all, Jesus Christ.  He instructed his disciples (Matthew 6: 5-13) to pray:

- privately to God without great show or fanfare
- simply and clearly, avoiding unnecessary wordiness and babbling
- with offerings of praise to God
- for the advancement of God's kingdom in this world
- for the provision of daily needs, recognizing that God best knows what those needs are
- for forgiveness and with a heart to forgive others
- for strength to recognize and resist temptation
- with acknowledgement that God is the ultimate power in all lives

There needn't be formality in prayer, but rather, a normal conversational style as though communicating with a friend (which you are to the Lord).  God isn't concerned with your eloquence but that you are coming to Him.  You can compare it to the way parents feel when their children come to them with an honest, open expression of feelings and concerns.  The parents are touched by their children's heart, not the sophistication of their communication style, and delight in the fact that their children love and trust them sufficiently to seek their advice and assistance. So too, God delights when His children seek his guidance and help.

There can be a variety of intents to your prayer.  Prayers of *thanksgiving* offer praise to the Lord for His creation, His presence, and for dying for your sins.  Prayers of *intercession* enable you to express your love for others---your family members, ministers, missionaries, government leaders, warring nations, the troubled-looking teen behind the counter at the fast-food restaurant---by lifting their needs to God.  Prayers for *healing* show your faith that the Lord can bring comfort, peace, and purpose in the midst of physical and emotional suffering.  Prayers for *forgiveness* of your sin help you to maintain a short account with God and clears the path from obstacles that could interfere with the experience of a full relationship with the Lord.  Prayers for God's *guidance* reflect your dependence on the Lord for the decisions and actions facing you as you live your life.

Meditating on Scripture as part of prayer can deepen communication with God and offer profound insights.  It is remarkable how God can speak if you take the time to listen.

Leanne Payne in her book *Listening Prayer*[9] describes practices that hinder prayer.  She cautions against the "disease of introspection" that causes us to sink into self-analysis during prayer time whereby we focus on ourselves rather than God.  Substitution is another hindrance and occurs when we pray to take on another person's pain or troubles, thereby becoming the savior-redeemer rather than allowing God to assume His rightful role.  Focusing on fighting demons and praying against Satan also hinders prayer as it distracts us from the focus of our prayers---God.

It is useful for you to dedicate a specific time of day for prayer.  Like any other practice, establishing a routine increases the likelihood that prayer becomes a habit.  In addition, you can engage in short prayer throughout the day.  These short prayers can relate to issues included in your routine prayer time or issues that surface as you go about your daily activities.  For example, you may pray that:

- you be helped to show patience and grace with the less than polite drivers on the highway
- you adopt a servant's heart rather than complain about the dishes left in the sink
- you be guided to make the best decision regarding how to respond to an invitation from a neighbor who you think you have nothing in common with
- the person in the ambulance that passes you receive the care needed in a timely manner

Your deep, routine prayers help to knit a strong fabric of relationship with God that covers you as you face life's challenges.  In addition, your short incidental prayers provide patches that reinforce the areas of life subjected to greater stress and prevent frayed fragments from tearing apart the basic fabric of a Christian walk.


## Study

My father became employed as a bricklayer for Bethlehem Steel Company after his discharge from the Navy. He had intentions of working there long enough to accumulate some money and return to college.  A growing family and pay incentives diverted his plans, and he spent the next 41 years laying brick inside blast furnaces.  The basic bricklaying skills he learned as an apprentice were sufficient to guide his career, and he was not required nor did he care to attend continuing education courses or read books about bricklaying. There was only so much one could learn about bricks and mortar.

Unlike laying brick, life as a Christian is not repetition of the same experience,  Rather, it requires that you be a lifelong student.  Even if you memorize the Bible from cover to cover, you will not reach a point in which you will know everything you need to know and have perfected the skills required to carry you through life's challenges.  You will encounter new challenges that you'll need to understand from a Biblical perspective, your mind and spirit will need regular nourishment, and your relationship with God will be a dynamic one in which He continues to teach you.

The Bible is the most important book to study---not merely read and hear, but really *study*. Studying implies that you are truly delving in and exploring the meaning of the words, reflecting on them, and thinking about what they mean for you. With this approach, you could spend days contemplating a single verse. For example, in studying the verse *Give us today our daily bread* (Matthew 6:11), you could sit with the verse for awhile, say it over and over, and ask God for insights. Consider what is meant by *daily bread*---ample food to nourish your body, the beauty of creation to nourish your soul, work to enable you to pay your bills, a loving spouse to lend support, the physical, emotional, and spiritual strength to face the challenges of the day. Reflect on the meaning of depending on God for daily provisions and God's reasons for wanting you to pray for daily provisions. Meditate on this and examine your attitude and behaviors in regard to this. Do you say you depend on God but feel that you still must take steps to assure you have a nest egg just in case His idea of provision isn't the same as yours? Is your daily bread based on true needs or desires for luxuries that you've become convinced that you need? Are you uncomfortable with the reality implicit in this verse? Studying this single verse could open the path to a lesson into your own heart and reveal areas that need prayer and work. True study of Scripture focuses on thoughtful examination of the words and their application, not just on reading a large number of pages; it is about quality, not quantity.

In addition to the Bible, there are other fine books that can be used for study. A visit to your local or online Christian bookstore can reveal the variety of topics to explore, such as study guides for specific books of the Bible, classical writings, contemporary issues, and guides for parenting, marriage, dating, and other aspects of living.

Group study can provide rich opportunities for learning. Many churches offer Bible study classes. BSF (Bible Study Fellowship International) is an interdenominational lay organization that offers classes throughout the world for men, women, and children; for the location in your community you may visit their website at www.bsfinternational.org or call 1-877-273-3228. If you're having difficulty finding a Bible study you may want to consider forming a group yourself in your neighborhood or over the lunch table at work. There are many easy-to-use study guides and books that include study questions that can be used to lead a group study.

Retreats can complement daily Bible study and provide an intense study time. Free from daily distractions, you may find you are able to concentrate more fully and spend longer blocks of time in uninterrupted contemplation. In addition to retreats sponsored by groups, you also can schedule your own private retreat. I know of mothers of young children who exchange weekend babysitting so that each one can enjoy a retreat while knowing their children are being well-cared for---without burdening the family budget. My husband and I have combined some of our vacation time together with private retreat time by staying at a site that provides outdoor areas or space within the hotel where we can get away from each other for blocks of time; after a full day of solitude and study, we reconnect for the evening. Think creatively as to the model that can work for you.

Self-study is a valuable exercise. It can be quite beneficial to periodically take stock of your life---your habits, your concerns, your reactions, burdens, and the people or events that influence you. Consider factors that could be contributing to your problems. You may find the core issues are that you are not in touch with God or that you've been straying from the Word.

Being attentive to the world around you is another important aspect of study. Allow your senses to study and experience the beauty of creation---the layers of feathers on a bird, the delicate petals on a flower, the scent of newly mowed grass, the sensation of raindrops against your face. Study the people around you to see how God is moving in their lives and lessons you can learn from them. Study the culture also. There is a risk that you may become so entwined in your Christian circle---socializing with Christian friends, listening to Christian music, reading Christian literature---that you are not aware of the activities and trends within society that could pose a threat to you, your family, and the church. Further, you may be more able to love and influence a person who doesn't know Christ if you've spent the time to understand that individual and the influences in his or her life.

Be a lifelong disciple!


## Fasting

Although discussed in detail earlier, it is beneficial to reinforce the importance of fasting. Secular health advocates promote the health benefits of fasting, yet Christians need to remember that fasting has been a spiritual discipline for as far back as can be remembered. Jesus' instructions on fasting begin with *"When you fast…"* (Matthew 6:16), implying that this was an expected practice for those who followed Christ.

You may think of fasting in terms of the omission of food; however, fasting from sinful behavior also must be considered. In her personal journals, Catherine Marshall[10], a gifted storyteller and wife of a former U. S. Senate Chaplain, describes how she attempted to fast from having a critical spirit for one day. This proved to be a challenge as she came to understand how automatic this behavior had become. During the day of fasting from critical behavior, God helped her to understand the fruitlessness of her ways and the extent to which it had blocked relationships and creativity. Convicted of her behavior, she was able to seek forgiveness and seek a new path. Be it criticism, sarcasm, nagging, gossiping, or other behaviors that separate us from positive, full relationships with God and others, fasting from sinful behaviors can aid in breaking our chains to them.

Fasting helps to keep balance in your life and prevents nonessential food, activities, stimulation, and other temptations from diverting your focus from the Lord. The self-denial experienced through fasting is a clear reminder that you must die to self to follow Jesus Christ; He is the subsistence of your life. The space that is emptying by that from which you fast can be filled by God's presence. Dallas Willard puts it well when he says "In fasting, we learn how to suffer happily as we feast on God[11]."

You may want to revisit the discussion of fasting in the chapter, Acquire Healthy Habits.

## Meditation

In secular holistic health circles, meditation is a popular practice that is widely promoted as a means to reduce stress, boost immunity, enhance clarity of thinking, and achieve a host of other benefits.  Eastern or transcendental meditation commonly is the model promoted and this form encourages deep relaxation with an emptying of the mind.  If any focus for the mind is suggested, it is on breathing patterns or a mantra.  In addition to the health benefits, "spiritual enlightenment" is considered a potential outcome in which the state of altered consciousness derived through the meditation potentially enables one to communicate with spiritual guides.  Obviously, this type of meditation poses problems for Christians in that it risks leaving our minds open to spiritual influences that may be demonic and assumes that we can rely on our own inner selves to achieve spiritual enlightenment.  I have encountered many Christians who carry such concerns about meditation and for these reasons they've rejected the practice altogether.

There is a place for meditation in the lives of Christians, and it is an important discipline.  In fact, the Bible shows evidence of this practice:

*He (Isaac) went out to the field one evening to meditate*  Genesis 24:63

*Do not let this Book of the Law depart from your mouth; meditate on it day and night…*  Joshua 1:8

*But his delight is in the law of the Lord, and on his law he meditates day and night*  Psalm 1:2

*My eyes stay open through the watches of the night, that I may meditate on your promises.*  Psalm 119:148

*…we take captive every thought to make it obedient to Christ*  2 Corinthians 10:5

There certainly are health benefits associated when Christians meditate, but most important is the closer relationship with God that can result.  Meditation as a spiritual discipline doesn't empty the mind but rather, focuses it on God and everything about Him.  When the mind is quieted, we often are able to gain insights from God and achieve greater union with Him.

Meditation can be a challenging discipline to practice because we live in a society that encourages and rewards us for our *doing* rather than our *being*.  Multitasking…improving efficiency and productivity… high-speed internet.  We constantly are bombarded with messages on how we can do more, faster.  In the midst of this climate, the act of sitting still and "doing nothing" can seem like a waste of time.  Yet, it can be critical to helping us to define ourselves by God's standards, not the world's, and draw us into a closer relationship with Him.

Although it is the substance not the mechanics of meditation that is important, there are some factors that can enhance the experience:

- Find a quiet, peaceful setting.  Some people find that sitting in a garden or near a body of water facilitates meditation.  However, if you don't have access to peaceful natural settings, you can create your own "sacred space" for meditating by placing some potted plants, candles, and religious objects on a table and instilling scents (aromatherapy) in the room.  Peaceful background music can be beneficial, also.
- Sit in a comfortable position; a lotus pose is not essential but sitting can be superior to lying down to assure you don't drift to sleep.
- Close your eyes and breathe deeply.  As you inhale, think about bringing in God's light and love; as you exhale release to God those thoughts that trouble or tempt you.

- Ask God to help you to stay focused on Him and to protect this time that you desire to be with Him.
- Think about an attribute of God, a Scripture verse, a recent experience in which you saw God work in your life, a lesson He has taught you.
- Be still and listen for God to speak to you. He speaks differently to different people. His voice may come through clearly in your mind, you may get a "sense" of a direction to take, or you suddenly think of a solution to a problem that has been plaguing you. Give Him time to communicate.
- If distractions (telephones, doorbells) or thoughts (I forgot to pick up milk, I wonder if the kids made a mess) invade your experience, take a deep breath and reorient yourself to meditating.

Some people find it useful to journal after meditating to record insights gained.

The act of meditation can promote the development of a meditative state of mind---i.e., being present in the moment---that permeates even the most common aspects of your daily life. You can become more attuned to the here and now, and control the extent to which distractions divert your attention. You can notice God's gifts in a renewed way. Examples of simple exercises to increase the art of being present in the moment include:

- Place a raisin in your palm. Examine all the ridges, the shape, the color of the fruit. Roll it between your fingers and feel the texture. Smell the raisin and then place it on your tongue. Roll it on your tongue, feeling the texture and size. Slowly chew the raisin and taste its flavor.
- Find a leaf that has fallen to the ground or pick one from a tree. Examine the color and shape, noticing changes from one section of the leaf to another. Gently stroke both sides of the leaf. Crush it in your hand and be aware of the feeling. Hold the pieces of the leaf to your nose and detect any scent that is present. Toss the pieces of the leaf in the air and watch them settle to the ground.

Simple acts such as these can help you to become more sensitive to the beauty and complexity of God's creation. The development of a meditative state of mind can help you to stay in touch with God throughout your daily routines, still your racing mind so that you keep stress under control, and maintain balance in your life.

## Solitude

Solitude was discussed in the chapter *Learn To Be Healthy* as a means to manage stress. Like meditation, this practice, although having health benefits, most importantly is a spiritual discipline that deepens our relationship to God. The need for time alone, apart even from those He loved, was demonstrated by Jesus:

*When Jesus heard what had happened, he withdrew by boat privately to a solitary place.* Matthew 14:13

*After he had dismissed them, he went up on a mountainside by himself to pray.* Matthew 14:23

*Very early in the morning, while it was still dark, Jesus got up, left the house and went off to a solitary place, where he prayed. Mark 1:35*

*But Jesus often withdrew to lonely places and prayed.* Luke 5:6

The solitude experienced as a spiritual discipline is not loneliness as you are engaging with the Lord during this time. In silence, you can have a vibrant, intimate conversation with God.

In addition to periods of solitude (e.g., several days away), you can also find mini-opportunities to practice this discipline by refraining from speech and interaction during the day. I know that personally, it is difficult for me to arrange a weekly day of solitude; however, I do find that I can build some solitude into each day by my habit of rising early and using that early morning time to contemplate on the Lord. You may find that you can schedule a short break between your arrival home and the beginning of household responsibilities to retreat to a corner of your home where your privacy will be respected, and you can have some quiet time with the Lord. You can achieve a state of solitude while sitting in traffic or on a bus as you block out the hustle-bustle around you and reflect on God and His creation. Although it is ideal to have a physical space where you can be alone for a period of time, when this is not possible, you can create a psychological and spiritual space to achieve oneness with God wherever you are.

## Self-Love

*So God created man in his own image…* Genesis 1:27

What an absolutely profound thought that we are made in the image of God…His likeness… a reflection of Him. We are His living, breathing representations on earth. Scripture offers many examples of our worth to God. The psalmist proclaims that God made us only *a little lower than heavenly beings and crowned us with glory and honor* (Psalm 8:5). Jesus tells us that every sparrow is remembered by God and since we are worth more than many sparrows, we have nothing to fear (Luke 12:6-7). We hold great value to God and to honor and love His creation of our being is to honor and love Him as the creator.

The apostle Paul advises to *love our neighbor as ourselves* (Romans 13:9). You must love yourself in order to understand how to love others and share God's love. One of the obstacles to the ability to fully love yourself could rest in the emotional baggage you carry regarding your shortcomings, failures, and sin. Consider Dave's example:

*Ten years ago, while on a business trip, Dave and a few of his associates decided to meet in the hotel lounge for a few drinks to celebrate the closing of a contract. After several rounds of drinks, Dave spotted what he believed to be the most gorgeous woman he had seen in a long time sitting at a table with some other women. Although married, Dave's inhibitions were significantly relaxed and he asked the object of his attention to dance. After a little playful objection, the woman conceded.*

*Dave learned that the woman's name was Elissa, and that she was married with two small children. Dave and Elissa shared several more dances and drinks, and began to confide how their marriages were unfulfilling. Before they knew it they exchanged a kiss, and then proceeded to Dave's hotel room where they both experienced their first affair.*

*The following morning, Dave's sense of excitement overcame the feelings of guilt he felt about his transgression. He believed he experienced things he hadn't felt in a long time. "This woman is my soul mate," he thought. "I've got to be with her."*

*The next several months were a whirlwind of rendezvous. The two met every chance they could. It was as though Dave wore special lenses that highlighted all the wonderful things about Elissa while exaggerating every fault of his wife. Less than four months after meeting, Dave and Elissa left their spouses and moved in together, over the objections and pleadings of their respective families.*

*This was the boldest things Dave had ever done in his life. He was usually responsible and level-headed, but he threw reason to the wind and followed his feelings. His wife had suspected nothing and was shocked that the life to which she was committed was crumbling before her. Dave still remembers the sick feeling in his stomach as he packed his things in his car and watched her sobbing uncontrollably and his little boy screaming, "Daddy, don't go." Although he had some thoughts that perhaps he was making a mistake, Dave knew Elissa had left her husband to be with him and felt that he had gone too far to turn back now.*

*The first year after leaving his wife was almost surreal. The worlds Dave and Elissa had known were destroyed as few friends and family associated with them. Elissa's children who now lived with Dave and Elissa, were acting out due to having their lives uprooted. Financial pressures mounted as Dave faced responsibility for two families.*

*Dave sensed some yellow lights in his relationship with Elissa, but ignored them, believing things would work out and that he had to accept his lot. Despite knowing problems existed in the relationship, Dave married Elissa as soon as their divorces were final. Within a year Elissa was pregnant. Dave was resentful as he trusted Elissa to faithfully use birth control. "The last thing I need is more expenses," he thought. Shortly after their first child together was born, they had a second, then a third child.*

*What had once been an exciting, passionate relationship now was burdensome and stressful. There never seemed to be enough money and Elissa never seemed to miss an opportunity to remind Dave of this, particularly as her first husband had become extremely successful in his business. The couple's sexual relationship felt more like an act of duty than an act of love. The kids complained that they couldn't afford the same things as their friends. Dave's son from his first marriage resented that he got less of his father's attention and resources than his father's new children.*

*Dave began to feel that he was reaping the results of his sin. He had committed adultery, caused the break-up of two families, hurt innocent people, made a mess of many lives. He reacted by withdrawing and becoming hostile. The slightest mishap or comment could set off a violent reaction that caused him to be physically and verbally abusive to anyone in his path. In the valley of self-hatred in which he lived, Dave could not truly love others.*

There is no ignoring the reality that Dave sinned when he betrayed his wedding vows; his adultery was wrong. Further, choosing the path of compounding his wrongs instead of repenting and returning to a right path added to his troubles. Imagine how differently Dave's life could have unfolded if after that first night in the hotel he had confessed his sin to his wife and God; asked both of them for forgiveness; asked Elissa for forgiveness; urged Elissa to set things right with her husband and God; sought Christian counseling; and prayed for guidance and strength. The Lord wants you to come to Him to repent and receive His forgiveness. *If we confess our sins, He is faithful and just and will forgive us our sins and purify us from all unrighteousness* (1 John 1:9). You can be cleansed and replace your guilt with His love. And, with an overflowing cup of His love, you will be able to love yourself and others more fully.

## Study Questions

1. What are some obstacles to prayer?  How can they be overcome?
2. What are some of the pros and cons of "studying" secular behaviors and trends?
3. Which of the spiritual disciplines discussed in this chapter are particularly challenging for you to practice?  Why?  What can you do to increase their presence in your life?
4. What unresolved sins of your past prevent you from loving yourself?  How can you relieve this burden?

## Related scriptures to pray

Deuteronomy 5:1
Psalm 119: 12-16, 23-24, 33-34
Proverbs 10:8
     23:12
     25:12
Matthew 4:4
     6: 5-13
     6:16-18
     24:41
John 8:32
Romans 8:6
     12:1
1 Corinthians 7:5
2 Corinthians 5:17
Philippians 4:6
Colossians 1:13
1 Thessalonians 5:17
1 John 1:7-2:2
2 Peter 1:5-8
     3:18

# CHAPTER 7
# CONNECT WITH OTHERS

God is a relational being and demonstrates this in a variety of ways. He exists in perfect relationship to the universe and Himself. He operates through a Trinity. Rather than a single human, He created a man and woman to multiply and live in community. Despite the ability to do anything He wants independent of us, He works through His people. Worshiping in community, loving one another, serving, and being other-centered are virtues He desires for us.

As God is connected to us, He so also desires that we connect with one another. *"Sure,"* you may say, *"I am around people all day. I see dozens of people at work, bump elbows with dozens more at the cafeteria, can barely find space to walk in the mall, and have kids running about the house most of the day."* Although you may come in contact with many people during the course of your day, you actually may not be connecting with them.

To a large extent, our society promotes separatism and individualism. I certainly confess to seeing many examples of this in my own life. My husband and I live on several acres in a comfortable-sized home. Months can pass before neighbors have occasion to see one another. I shop at several different supermarkets (depending on where I happen to be driving at the time!) where I seldom know the clerks. Voice mails have allowed me to exchange multiple messages without actually having to speak to a living being, and the internet has enabled me to conduct considerable activity with no human contact. I can amuse myself with computer games that I can play solo and enjoy movies in the comfort and privacy of my own livingroom.

I contrast my lifestyle to my parents'. They lived in an inner city rowhouse in a Greek community where neighbors not only knew each other, but usually knew what village others came from "in the Old Country." It was not unusual to see several generations living under one roof. If a neighbor was sick, lost a job, or had a fight with a spouse, word quickly spread and you could rest assured that someone would be visiting that household to offer help or advice. I knew that I'd better be on good behavior when outside my home as the other adults in the community wouldn't hesitate to correct me as though I belonged to them. When it rained and someone had clothes hanging on the line, the nearest neighbor would take them down if the lady of the house was out; the neighbor also would go in and close any opened windows because no one locked their doors. My mother shopped at the local grocery store that had been operated by the same family for decades. If my friends and I were short of change to pay for our purchases at the local drug store, the pharmacist, who knew us since we were carried in our mothers' arms, would tell us just to make it good the next time we came in. There were many "characters" whose peculiarities and flaws seasoned the atmosphere, but who were tolerated---and cared for. When the weather allowed, the most popular form of recreation was sitting in the back yard or on the front steps where the neighborhood adults would share news and life stories, and the kids would play catch, jacks, and dodge ball. I'm not claiming that this life was free of problems, but there was a richness to living in community. Although it can be more challenging for us than previous generations, a balanced life demands that we experience the richness of healthy connections.

## Reflecting on Your Life Story

Examining the significant people and events that shaped your life aids in understanding yourself and others. One means to accomplish this is to trace your life story. Writing your story helps you to clarify thoughts and reflect on your experiences, and also provides a record for you to leave for future generations. Also, by connecting the dots of your life journey you are able to see the various times and ways that God has appeared in your life.

Table 11 provides an outline of some of the historical events in your life that you may want to consider when recording your life story, although there certainly are other approaches that you can take. However, don't be discouraged if writing is a challenge for you. There are other means to document your life story, as is exemplified by Doris, a friend of mine:

*Doris has lived a vibrant Christian life for over six decades and had rich life experiences that ran the full continuum of good and bad, righteous and sinful, gut-wrenching and joyful. Her own difficulties and lessons, coupled with a love for the Lord and His people, led her to develop a lay counseling ministry in which the sharing of life stories helps people to learn, grow, and heal.*

*Through the years, many people who have heard Doris' story urged her to write it, believing it had the elements of a fascinating book. Unfortunately, Doris despised writing, despite knowing that her experiences could minister to others who could learn from her journey. Finally, a friend found the solution and convinced Doris to spend a few days at the beach where they could videotape Doris' story. It worked! Doris unfolded her life story as her friend, armed with her camcorder, recorded and guided her with key questions. Her friend then reviewed the tapes and typed the highlights, providing Doris a document from which to work.*

Don't be surprised if reflecting on your life stirs emotions---some of which may be uncomfortable. Surfacing and facing some of the lingering pain, resentments, guilt, and unfinished business may be necessary in order to move ahead. Ask the Lord to reveal aspects of your life that continue to limit your ability to live abundantly and for guidance on how they can be addressed. Review of your life story can not only surface uncomfortable feelings, though. There can be tremendous joy in reminiscing about your childhood or special---and even ordinary---experiences in your life. You may realize that a friend or relative has woven a thread through your life in a special way, coming to your aid when needed or showing you different facets of life; this awareness could stimulate you to express your appreciation to that individual. Recognizing the obstacles you've overcome, you may take delight in your blessings.

---

**Table 11**
**Suggested Content for Your Life Story**

Family background
- Description of parents, grandparents, significant relatives
- Siblings
- Religious and spiritual beliefs and practices

Childhood
- Birth: where, when, unusual events
- Reasons you were given your name
- Favorite activities, interests
- School
- Friends
- Family dynamics
- Special experiences
- Unpleasant experiences
- Relationship with God, religious activities

Adolescence
- Favorite activities, interests
- School
- Friends; role/position in peer group
- Family dynamics
- Special experiences
- Unpleasant experiences
- Relationship with God, religious activities

Adulthood
- Reasons for career choice
- Various jobs you've held
- Education
- When, how, where you met your spouse
- Feelings about marriage
- Where you've lived
- Family dynamics
- Friends
- Favorite activities, interests
- Special experiences
- Unpleasant experiences
- Relationship with God, religious activities, spiritual growth
- Ways in which God has acted in your life
- Legacy you'd like to leave

---

## Relationships

After you've explored the threads that have woven the tapestry of your life, you may be better equipped to sew healthy relationships with others. As mentioned, God is relational and wants us to be in dynamic relationship with others. Through relationships, we show God's love and see His love manifested in a variety of ways. The proof that God knows what is best for us is reflected in various studies that have demonstrated higher levels of health and improvements in health conditions when individuals are engaged in loving, supportive relationships (e.g., married people have lower suicide rates than those who are alone; married men live longer than single men). Good relationships can teach, encourage, inspire, expand, and restore us.

Examine your relationships. Jesus commanded us to love one another and you may want to consider if your interactions with others reflect this. It can be helpful to create an image in your mind of echoes and mirrors when you think about your relationships in that what you get back depends on what you give. Remember the wise advice offered in Scripture:

*As I have loved you, so you must love one another* John 13:34

*Love your enemies* Matthew 5:34

*A friend loves at all times* Proverbs 17:17

*Do not judge* Matthew 7:1

*Do not take revenge* Romans 12:19

*If someone strikes you on the right cheek, turn to him the other also* Matthew 5:39

*Whoever loves God must also love his brother* 1John 4:21

Jesus wants you to show love, forgiveness, acceptance, and tolerance in your relationships, yet that does not mean you must allow yourself to be subjected to the abusive, destructive, or sinful behaviors of others. When you are faced with these situations some useful measures could include:

- *Examining your role.* Consider what you may be communicating through your words and actions---and through what you do not say and do---that could be giving the other person an incorrect message. For example, if you have a friend who repeatedly tells her spouse that she is spending time with you when she actually is spending that time engaging in an adulterous relationship, and expects that you'll cover for her, examine what message you have conveyed that could have been interpreted as your acceptance of this arrangement. You may not like to be placed in this situation but are uncomfortable confronting your friend; perhaps you said "Well, you know this isn't right, but okay, just this time"; or maybe you've inadvertently encouraged the relationship by making comments such as "He does seem like a nice person."
- *Praying.* Ask the Lord to reveal the truth and guide you in doing what is right. He often can show paths to correcting a bad situation that you alone couldn't have considered.
- *Seeking counsel.* Discuss the matter with your pastor or another mature Christian who can offer insights and lead you to helpful Scripture.
- *Confronting the matter.* Ignoring unhealthy or sinful actions that impact you serves no purpose. Discuss the issue with the individual, kindly and gently. Rather than attack the person with judgmental statements (e.g., "You'll go to hell for treating me so badly." "You're a horrible sinner." "God hates you for what you're doing."), present the issue from the perspective of how you feel (e.g., "It hurts me when you treat me this way," "I feel uncomfortable being asked to lie for you as I

believe it is the wrong thing to do," "I care for you as a friend and it grieves me to see you committing adultery.") Be direct.

- *Offering paths to changing the situation.* Provide suggestions for resources (e.g., Christian counseling, support groups, AA, etc.) that can assist. Pray for and offer to pray with the person. Ask the person for insights and suggestions that can aid in the resolution.

Table 12 offers some suggestions for healthy relationships.

---

### Table 12    Suggestions for Healthy Relationships

- Treat each person as though he or she was Jesus.
- Tame your tongue and think before you speak.
- Choose to love rather than be driven by feelings.
- Offer time for responses and reactions to surface.
- Put others first.
- Be hospitable and find ways to serve others.
- Be humble.
- Avoid judgmental behavior and revenge; repay evil with love and good deeds.
- Honor commitments.
- Foster peace and harmony.
- Appreciate diversity in attributes, giftedness, behaviors.
- Communicate assertively.
- Resolve conflict in a win-win manner.
- Speak about feelings rather than judgments.
- Present complaints in the form of suggestions or requests.
- Show grace and give the benefit of the doubt.
- Take time to reflect and understand.
- Forgive and move on.
- Know when to prune relationships.
- Encourage, empower, and build up others.
- When faced with difficult situations in relationships, refer to the Bible to see what Jesus did in these circumstances.
- Respect others, remembering each are God's children.

---

*Marriage*

The marriage relationship is a very special and sacred one. It also can be among the more challenging of the relationships experienced, particularly in the 21st Century when the message from the secular world implies that the Biblical model for a marital relationship is irrelevant and even oppressive. Same sex marriages and parenting increasingly are accepted as legitimate options to the traditional nuclear family model. In some circles, the concept of wives submitting to husbands as head of the family is viewed as highly distasteful and demeaning to women.  Celebrities who birth babies out of wedlock are glamorized while couples who commit to Godly principles of childrearing get little attention.

I must confess to sharing society's critical views of marriage during the early part of my adult life, before becoming a Christian.  I entered adulthood during the rise of feminism when "women can have it all" seemed to be the mantra.  The stay-at-home mom families I had seen often reflected women frustrated by boredom and underutilized gifts, and husbands who ran the extremes of abusive tyrants to detached paycheck providers.  Marriage was fine as long as everyone *felt good* within it; if it was no longer fulfilling or if a better catch caught one's eye, a marriage could be broken and one could move on to greener pastures.  Despite tracking in many circles and having many friends and acquaintances, no one ever shared the Biblical model for marriage.  It wasn't until midlife that I learned about God's plan for marriage and the blessings it held.  I can't help but wonder if many other people are misguided because Christians haven't come into their paths and boldly shared the realities and virtues of Biblical manhood and womanhood.

So, what does the Bible tell us about marriage?
- God created man and woman to be in relationship and multiply (Genesis 1:27-28; 2:18).  He could have chosen to let Adam rule alone or to provide a same sex partner to rule with Adam, yet God created two different sexed beings to complement each other and reproduce.
- Marriage is a sacred act that is a dynamic reflection of Christ and the Church (Ephesians 5:23-33).
- Being created in the image of God, both sexes are equal in worth (Genesis 1:26; 1Peter 2:17).  They both have been redeemed by Jesus Christ
- The husband is the head of his wife (Genesis 2:15-25; Ephesians 5:22-33; 1Corinthians 11:3).  This headship does not imply male dominance, but rather, the husband leading, protecting and loving his wife as Christ did in his authority over the Church.
- The wife is to submit to her husband and be his helpmate (Genesis 2:18; Ephesians 5:22-33; 1Corinthians 11:3).  This does not suggest that the woman is inferior to the man, but that they have distinctly different and complementary roles within the family.  It is interesting to note that in the Hebrew text, helper does not imply subordination but usually is used in context of God helping and serving others.
- Marriage is intended to be lasting (Matthew 19:6).  Jesus made it clear that He did not condone finding reasons to divorce, but in committing to a lasting relationship.
- Marriage is to be filled with joy, romance, and intimacy, as a creation of God (Song of Songs).

It is no secret that God's principles for a holy marriage cause interesting reactions in society that often can create challenges for Christians.  Audrey's example is a case in point.

*Audrey and Bill met in high school and experienced an immediate attraction.  Despite attending colleges in different states, their relationship deepened.  They both were committed Christians and shared similar values.*

*Following college graduation they married.  They both continued their education while working part-time and in a few years, Bill became a CPA and Audrey obtained a law degree and passed the bar. A bright and dynamic couple, they supported each other's careers.*

*After a few years of marriage, the couple was blessed with a daughter. Audrey had stopped working during her last month of pregnancy and stayed at home with her child until she entered first grade. At that time, with her husband's enthusiastic support, Audrey decided to return to work, part-time. The stimulation was welcomed, as was the extra money that came in handy for her daughter's private school. She was able to take cases that afforded her a schedule that allowed her to be home when her daughter left and returned from school; however, even with a part-time schedule she found it challenging to cook homemade meals and keep a tidy house. Bill pitched in as he could, but the housekeeping standards within their home were considerably more relaxed than before she returned to work.*

*It didn't take long for Audrey to begin feeling that she fit into neither the professional world nor the mommy world. Colleagues would question how she could let her investment in her career be underutilized by taking "Mickey Mouse cases" and not participating in activities for professional advancement. Her stay-at-home friends would ask her if she felt her family was suffering because her time and energy were being shared with a job; there was an implication that working outside the home was improper for a Christian wife and mother. Audrey began to feel that she was a foreigner in both lands, and even worse, that perhaps she was being an ungodly wife and mother.*

Audrey's dilemma is not an uncommon one. Many feminists would balk at a woman forfeiting her career to stay at home to care for husband, home, and children. And on the other hand, many Christians would criticize a woman who chose to work outside the home. Certainly, a mother's presence with a child during the early years of life is significant to the child's optimal development; no day care arrangement is superior to the nurturing provided by a loving parent. Attending to the physical, emotional, and spiritual well-being of one's child is a demonstration of good stewardship of this blessing from the Lord. However, God has not forbid women from having gainful employment outside the home. In fact, a review of the attributes of the Proverbs 31 Wife of Noble Character demonstrates this in that she (Proverbs 31:10-31):

- works with eager hands
- brings food from afar
- provides food for her family
- considers a field, buys it, and works it
- sets about her work vigorously
- sees that her trading is profitable
- makes and sells linen garments
- watches over the affairs of her household
- does not eat the bread of idleness

In addition to providing useful services and assisting their families, women can be a light of the Lord in the workplace. They may have the chance to share the gospel and field questions with people who would not venture into a church, but who need to know the Lord. Work can be a ministry.

A working wife does create a different dynamic within the family. She seldom is able to do all of the nice little things that a stay-at-home wife can. The house may not be spic and span at all times and the cookie jar may lack homemade goodies.  Husbands and children may have to pick up household responsibilities that aren't at the top of their list of things they love to do.  And, there will be times when the woman comes home tired and stressed, not only unable to give a lot to others, but perhaps in need of some TLC herself.  Families need to address these issues realistically, pray for guidance, talk with couples who have faced both sides of the issue, and reach a consensus regarding the decision.  Without reaching a decision that both husband and wife can live with, tension and conflict in the marital relationship can result.

Work and childrearing styles are only two of the many critical issues couples will face in their marriage.  In-laws, pets, friends, money, leisure pursuits, church membership, and schedules are among the topics that can create conflict between even the most loving couples.  It can be useful for couples to learn about their partners' basic values that influence their attitudes and behaviors.  Table 13 offers an exercise that can be used to stimulate discussions between couples as to values differences that potentially could lead to conflict.  Christian premarital counseling and classes can provide valuable assistance to couples in gaining insights into potential areas of conflict and learning skills to resolving matters constructively.

## Table 13  Exploring Values in Relationships

*Directions:  Provide a copy of this list for both you and your partner.  Each of you circle 10 words on your list that reflect values that are most important. Compare your lists and discuss differences.*

| | |
|---|---|
| Achievement | Joy |
| Affluence | Love |
| Ambition | Marriage |
| Biblical conformity | Material possessions |
| Casualness | Obedience |
| Cautiousness | Openness |
| Career | Orderliness |
| Celebration | Patience |
| Change | Peace |
| Community | Perfection |
| Compassion | Perseverance |
| Competitiveness | Physical beauty |
| Consistency | Popularity |
| Creativity | Privacy |
| Effectiveness | Purity |
| Efficiency | Recognition |
| Environmental protection | Relaxation |
| Excellence | Respect |
| Excitement | Risk-taking |
| Extravagance | Routine |
| Faithfulness | Secrecy |
| Fame | Security |
| Family | Self-control |
| Fidelity | Self-fulfillment |
| Forgiveness | Sensitivity |
| Formality | Service |
| Freedom | Sexual gratification |
| Friendships | Silence |
| Frugality | Socialization |
| Fun | Solitude |
| Genuineness | Spiritual development |
| Growth | Spontaneity |
| High stimulation | Stability |
| Honesty | Success |
| Humor | Tolerance |
| Independence | Trust |
| Influence | Truth |
| Ingenuity | Work |
| Integrity | Worship |

*Parenting*

Children are a blessing from God and in that context, the relationship between parents and their children need to glorify God.  Parents are the worldly agents for God as they guide and train their children into the roles of godly men and women.  This implies that the goal isn't for parents to make children happy or be buddies with them, but rather, to serve their children responsibly by:

- guiding them in understanding that they are God's creation, each made for a unique purpose and possessing a full account of God's love
- exercising authority, setting limits, and disciplining when necessary
- teaching children how to discern and respond to the world in which they live
- helping them to understand not only the mistakes they make, but the underlying reason why the matter is wrong in God's eyes
- assisting and encouraging them to worship Jesus Christ rather than other idols (e.g., expensive clothes, cars, toys)
- demonstrating and asking for forgiveness
- offering opportunities for spiritual growth
- affording opportunities for quality recreational experiences that contribute to their spiritual development
- providing shaping influences within the home of love, service, order, grace, respect, honor to commitments, and reliance on God rather than worldly solutions
- practicing the same pure, unselfish love that God offers them

## Worship

In the broadest sense, to worship is to adore God and honor His worth.  Most of us tend to think of religious services within church buildings as worship, however, our praise, adoration, and celebration of the Lord ideally are integrated into our daily lives---not just reserved for Sunday mornings.  We worship God when we acknowledge that He is the creator of the sweet song the bird sings outside our window; when we treat the stranger we encounter in the mall with the same sensitivity that Jesus did when He met crowds in Galilee; when we take a pause from our daily routines to feel, *truly feel,* deep gratitude for the reality of Christ dying for our sins; and when we open our hearts and minds and invite the Lord to speak to us.  Regardless of the place or process, Jesus is the object of our worship.

An exciting connection with God and others can be achieved through the corporate worship experience. People who gather with the expectancy of dynamic interaction with God create a sacred space that allows God to be present.  The unity of multiple spirits has a synergy that surpasses the power of a single individual. Together they sing, pray, dance, and rejoice to praise him.  Their whole bodies engage with the Lord; their hearts and spirits are naked before Him.

It is important for you to find a house of worship in which you can achieve a sense of community.  Search for a church in which you can connect with others, comfortably participate, and focus on the worship experience.  This may mean that the church may not be the most convenient or elaborate building, but is one that facilitates a dynamic, interactive relationship with God.  It isn't the building that houses the worshipers that is important, but rather, the worship experience that is housed within the structure.

## Service

Deeds do not substitute for a vibrant relationship with Christ or a life lived according to God's will.  However, service is an important part of the Christian walk, reinforced by messages that we carry each other's burdens, and in this way we will fulfill the law of Christ (Galatians 6:2).  Jesus made it clear that this life isn't about self-centeredness and self-benefit but rather, denying ourselves and losing our lives for Him (Matthew 16:24-25).  In His greatness, He could have required that others serve Him, yet He provided the ideal model of the servant leader by washing His disciples' feet, feeding the hungry, healing the sick, and dying for our sins.

The discipline of service in a Christian's life is for the glorification of God, not for personal recognition and reward.  And, it is indiscriminate in that you do not choose to serve in situations that are necessarily fun and fulfilling for you.  Let me share two examples from a ministry in which I served.

*Northern Baltimore County Faith in Action was an interfaith volunteer caregiving ministry that provided emotional and spiritual support and chore assistance to elderly and disabled individuals.  It was an important ministry that offered opportunities for Christians to demonstrate their love for the Lord through service while providing assistance to persons who may otherwise not be able to receive the help and support they need.  On one occasion, a woman with grown children signed on to volunteer and was assigned to an older woman who needed someone to visit, run errands, and do minor chores that she no longer was able to do on her own.  After a few visits the volunteer phoned and asked if she could be reassigned.  "What is wrong?  Was there a problem?" I queried.  "Well, no, not exactly," she responded.  "It's just that this lady wasn't all that interesting, and she wanted me to do things like dust her furniture.  I don't even dust my own furniture," she exclaimed.*

*During this same time another volunteer, Andy, joined the ministry---a well-polished, energetic man with an active family, car dealership, and busy life.  He was assigned to visit a man who was quadriplegic and could do little else than talk.  The intent was to provide this disabled man with someone who could visit periodically and talk about "guy stuff."  The relationship unfolded into a very special one, and within in a short time, Andy was taking this wheelchair-bound man to baseball and football games, which required that he transport the gentleman in his special van, negotiate a wheelchair through crowded stadiums, and manage the special needs that arose during their time together.  Andy continued to make time and space in his life to visit this man regularly for years with few people having any idea of the wonderful act of service he was displaying.*

Andy had the heart of a servant in his volunteer experience.  He put the needs of the disabled man he served ahead of the personal inconvenience and sacrifice of time he could have been spending on other activities.  He didn't get embarrassed when he would draw stares as he pushed his wheelchair-bound friend in public places.  He didn't care that he was investing time and energy in something that didn't advance his economic or personal status, or even provide some pleasure for himself.  He wasn't at all concerned that few people seemed to know of his volunteerism.  Andy has a servant's  heart and serves as he is called---not for himself, but for the Lord.

What does it take to have a servant's heart?  It is an attitude, a way of being.  A servant is:
- interested in the needs of others
- empathetic
- open to learning about others
- a good listener
- willing to sacrifice time, energy, resources
- a good steward of the gifts and talents with which he or she has been blessed
- committed to the kingdom of Christ

A Christian demonstrates a servant's heart in every domain of life---family, church, work, and play.  In some circumstances, this may involve major actions, such as giving a large sum of money to a coworker whose house has been destroyed by fire or committing to a long-term mentoring relationship with a troubled teenager.  At other times, it can entail being a blessing to someone in a small way---such as carrying an extra workload on a day that a coworker is not feeling well or helping the young mother with several children carry her groceries to her car.

Being a servant tends to run counter to society's norms.  The not so subtle message conveyed through the popular media and lifestyles of those celebrated by the secular world is that *if it feels right for you, you have a right to do it.*  We witness examples of corporate raiders making millions of dollars while destroying the jobs of the average worker; celebrities having babies out of wedlock to satisfy their parental stirrings without consideration of the best interests of their children; political leaders violating their marital vows and the dignity of public office by having serial affairs.  In a climate of self-gratification, putting the needs of others ahead of oneself seems ludicrous.  Yet, loving others as much as we love ourselves is exactly what Christians are commanded to do.  It is one of the areas where the rubber meets the road in our Christian walk.

## Study Questions

1. If you could write the ideal obituary for yourself, what would it say?
2. If you are part of a couple, what 3 values do you and your partner most share and on what 3 values do you differ?
3. Why is it so difficult to tame the tongue?
4. What are your children's strengths and weaknesses?  What can you do to reinforce their strengths and correct their weaknesses?
5. What factors in society create challenges in developing and sustaining godly relationships?  What are some ways that theses challenges can be overcome?

## Related scriptures to pray

Genesis 50:19-21
Proverbs 9:7-10
       18:2
Matthew 4:10
       12:30
John 13:14
Colossians 3:19
Philippians 2:14
Ephesians 5:23-33
1John 4:21
James 1:19-20
      3: 1-18

# CHAPTER 8
# EXPERIENCE LIFE'S BLESSINGS

Taking care of the temple God has given you, using your spiritual gifts, and exercising the spiritual disciplines foster holistic health. Certainly this has many positive results for you, such as preventing illness, having ample energy to face the challenges of each day, and enjoying feelings of peace and well-being. Yet, your reasons for caring for your body, mind, and spirit are not just for your own personal benefit, but very importantly, to experience the Lord and His blessings more fully so that you can offer Him your best for His use.

## Purpose

God created you as a unique individual, with features, gifts, and talents that are tailor made for you. He desires you to use them to His glory, for the purpose of being more like Christ. The more you discover, develop, and use the unique attributes He has given you, the more you will learn about the person you were created to be and the ways in which you can conform to the Lord's likeness.

*What is your purpose?* Perhaps you haven't given this much thought, or maybe you define it by the priorities facing you at the time, such as being a parent, earning a living, or singing in the church choir. Certainly, purpose can be realized through these avenues, but it may be useful to consider if you are truly realizing *God's purpose* for you through these activities. Consider Jeff's example:

> *Having excelled in his graduate work, Jeff was being aggressively recruited by several major corporations by the time he finished his M.B.A. He accepted a position with a company that dangled the promise of a fast track up the corporate ladder, and true to their promise, the company rewarded Jeff's outstanding work by advancing him quickly. By his tenth year of employment, Jeff was a corporate vice president.*
>
> *During his corporate rise Jeff became married and had three children. He and his wife were both Christians who committed to having the Lord's presence in their lives. They were active in their church and assured that their children received a solid foundation for their Christian walk. Jeff felt blessed that he could afford to have his wife homeschool their children and that his income allowed him to give generously to the church---far beyond the expected tithe.*

*Jeff had become an elder in the church and significantly contributed to the church's organizational development through his business savvy. Although he committed his time and money to the church, Jeff was feeling some unrest. Despite his successful corporate career, there were stirrings within, that there was something more, something different intended for him. Jeff had no idea what this meant and attributed it to everything from an early midlife crisis to a need for some time off. He prayed for guidance and clarity.*

*It wasn't long after Jeff experienced these stirrings that the church hired a consultant to review their activities and offer recommendations. The church had experienced growth beyond its expectations and was facing the trials and tribulations of a growing organization. One of the major recommendations given by the consultant was that the church separate the administrative activities from the senior pastor's responsibilities and hire someone with a strong business background who could direct the church in strategic planning, fiscal management, personnel issues, and other administrative matters. "A seasoned Christian with a MBA would be an ideal candidate," the consultant commented during his exit conference with the elders. Jeff felt the eyes of the other elders look to him. Jeff never imagined that his stirrings could have meant this, and he wasn't sure how he felt about it. He recognized that he would be an ideal candidate for the job, yet he knew the church could pay nowhere near what he was making in corporate America; further, he wondered what this would mean to his career.*

*The church offered the job to Jeff and over the next few months he and his wife prayed on this issue. They knew the job change would mean less income, but rather than see the luxuries they would have to do without, they were able to rejoice at the blessings they were afforded by Jeff enjoying a decade of high earnings that allowed them to buy their home and accumulate a small savings. Jeff accepted the position and found the challenges, daily comradery with Christians, and the opportunity to further God's kingdom through his work, more than compensated for the difference in salary.*

Jeff discovered peace and fulfillment by accepting the call to fill God's purpose for him. Some people may question an executive forfeiting an impressive income and corporate power, and even charge that he isn't thinking about the best interest of his family. Yet, by following his call, Jeff is offering his family a priceless gift.

So, how can you know your purpose? Consider asking yourself what activities:

- express your reasons for existence?
- do you love to do?
- have been confirmed through prayer?
- you'd do whether or not you excelled, got paid, or received recognition?
- bring you a sense of peace?
- do you engage in that you can find Biblical examples of godly people engaging in?
- have brought about positive results confirmed by God?
- are God-glorifying and bring others closer to God?

It is important to understand that God can use brokenness, pain, and hardship to help you to achieve your purpose. Through hardships and weaknesses you can become more compassionate, pliable, and open to serving God. One only need to read the book of Job to appreciate this. Likewise, your purpose may not be readily apparent, and God may place you in various situations to prepare you for the purpose He has in mind for you. Consider the life of Joseph (Genesis 30-50):

*Joseph was bright, and of his father's, Jacob's, twelve sons, he was the favorite. With his self-assured air, he shared a dream in which he saw part of the vision God had for him, which included ruling over his brothers. His youthful immaturity led him to boast about the wonderful designs God had on his life, rather than to seek God's guidance and timing. Needless to say this fueled his brothers' jealousy and anger toward him. Although his brothers initially plotted to kill him, Joseph was spared from death and sold as a slave. This experience was part of God's molding of Joseph, and Joseph was put in charge of his master, Potiphar's, household, thereby providing him with the experience that he would need for the responsibilities in his future. However, there was another twist in his journey, as Potiphar's wife, angered by Joseph's rejection of her sexual advances, reported to her husband that Joseph had attempted to seduce her, resulting in Joseph being placed in prison.*

*Although Joseph probably had times when he scratched his head wondering what God was doing to him, he remained faithful. When he overheard the Pharaoh's chief cupbearer and baker discussing a dream, he interpreted it for them, using it as an experience to glorify the Lord rather than to promote his own talents. The soon to be freed cupbearer agreed to explain Joseph's innocence to the Pharaoh to assist in Joseph's release, yet failed to do so for two years. Still, Joseph trusted God and remained faithful.*

*Finally, an opportunity came for the cupbearer to tell the Pharaoh about Joseph when a dream interpreter was needed. Pharaoh was so impressed with Joseph's wisdom and discernment that he put him in charge of Egypt. In this position, Joseph was able to demonstrate his capabilities, saving the Israelites from famine. Through his reliance and faithfulness to God through what probably seemed like senseless ordeals, Joseph was able to be prepared for a significant leadership role that secured the survival of God's chosen people.*

Like Joseph, you too must be faithful and reliant on God, recognizing that everything that happens in your life is preparing you for your unique purpose.

Following God's purpose for you doesn't mean you need to avoid secular employment or take a vow of poverty. You can use your gifts in any setting or as part of ordinary daily activities. There are numerous examples of the way Jesus used opportunities to demonstrate purpose as part of ordinary life events. For example, He seized teachable moments with whoever was near Him and didn't wait until a strategically planned event was conducted to offer His wisdom. Rather than scheduling healing services at designated times and places, He healed those He encountered on His journey. Being part of Christ's living kingdom is to realize purpose wherever you happen to be at any time---often by living an ordinary life in an extraordinary manner.

## Celebration

I remember trying to speak to a nonbelieving relative about developing a relationship with Jesus Christ. As soon as he realized what I was talking about he stopped me and said, "Look, I may be interested in that stuff when I'm older, but now I'm in my prime and not ready to give up my good times." His reaction was similar to many people who believe that a decision to be a Christian implies a solemn, plain, and boring lifestyle. Unfortunately, the flames of this man's attitude have been fanned by people who call themselves Christians, but who are more focused on rules, rituals, and restrictions than a dynamic, authentic relationship with Jesus Christ.

There is nothing in the Bible that says you must forfeit pleasure and joy for God.  Quite the contrary!  He invites you to make a joyful noise unto Him, rejoice and be glad, and live an abundant life.  The Bible is sprinkled with examples of feasts and celebrations.  Paul proclaims that the kingdom of God is about righteousness, peace and *joy* in the Holy Spirit (Romans 14:17).  Joy often is commanded in the Bible:

*Sing joyfully to the Lord* (Psalm 33:1)

*Be joyful always* (1 Thessalonians 5:16)

*Rejoice in the Lord always.  I will say it again, Rejoice!* (Philippians 4:4)

In the rational, sophisticated, and achievement-oriented world in which you live, playfulness, joy, fun, and celebration may seem to be an afterthought or described as achievable only through the latest car, movie, or resort.  Yet, God wants you to have pleasure through a relationship with Him.  A joyless life hardly is a testimony to the Lord.

Celebration begins with a realization of your blessings.  Take a few minutes and think about the answers to these questions:

- What 3 blessings have you experienced in the past week?  (These can include simple things in your routine day, such as a friend taking your children on a day when you weren't feeling well.)
- What 3 blessings have you experienced in this past year?
- What major blessings can you recall when reflecting on your entire life?

You may be surprised to see that you have been blessed more than you realize.  Show your gratitude to the Lord by joyfully offering praise for these blessings.

It also is useful to reflect on those individuals who have touched your life and develop a written *gratitude list*.  List the way the person has blessed your life and then plan some ways that you can express your gratitude.  For example:

| Person | Blessing offered to me: | Plans to show my appreciation: |
| --- | --- | --- |
| *Aunt Irene* | *Patiently listened to me during times when I questioned God's existence*<br><br>*Regularly sent me inspirational books to mold my thinking* | *Send her a letter thanking her for her support and patience*<br><br>*Send her books that now inspire me with notes* |
| *Mom* | *Unconditional love*<br><br>*A secure and safe home* | *Tell her how much I appreciate her*<br><br>*Create a scrapbook of her life for each of her grandchildren so that they will know about this special lady* |
| *Nora, my neighbor* | *Does dozens of little things for me without fuss or fanfare* | *Plant a tree in Nora's backyard in honor of our friendship* |

Expressing gratitude is a form of celebration that enriches the hearts of others.

Find ways to make holidays a celebration to honor the Lord.  This may be less difficult for holidays such as Christmas and Easter than for some others.  Yet, there are many ways that a holiday occasion can be used to create an opportunity for fun, fellowship, and praise to God.  For example:

- *Presidents' Day*:  Host a pot luck dinner and game night.  Create your own game of trivia in which you give historical facts or characteristics of various leaders in the Bible and guests try to guess who is being described.
- *Independence Day:*  In addition to celebrating the independence of our country, why not organize role plays of Biblical characters who were freed from sin and burdens (e.g., Job, David, Joseph, Paul)?
- *Labor Day:*  Organize a group of friends and family to volunteer for a project (e.g., community clean-up, visit to a nursing home, planting a tree) topped off with a cookout to thank the Lord for the ability to work.
- *Halloween:*  Offer an alternative to secular celebrations by holding a feast to honor the special gifts of Fall.

The possibilities are endless.

You can also create celebrations to make ordinary days special.  My husband holds this wonderful memory of a "celebration" that his parents once created:

*George's family lived in a townhouse in a community of many children.  During a snowstorm, the neighborhood kids were eager to be playing outdoors but without open fields and hills, their options were somewhat limited.  In the midst of brainstorming with his friends on what they could do, George noticed his mother intently moving the snow about in their small backyard.  She leveled a large area and then began wetting it with the garden hose.  "What was she doing?" he wondered.  Not long thereafter, she called to him and his friends, "Hey guys, you want to skate?"  Although embarrassed by what he perceived as another one of his mother's crazy ideas, George couldn't help but notice that his friends took interest and began migrating to his backyard.  Before he knew it, the yard was packed with kids, skating, sliding, and slipping on the makeshift ice rink, having a ball.  George's father then set up the grill and cooked hotdogs.  Neighbors, seeing the activity, came with cookies, pots of hot chocolate, and whatever else they had to share.  The creativity shown by George's mother led to an unplanned celebration that resulted in a special bonding of neighbors… and a warm memory that remains with her children long after her death.*

The nourishment of the spirit through the act of celebration gives strength to life and enables you to put events in perspective.  It is a proactive means to instill wholesome fun into life.  Without this, a void can exist which could be filled by Satan.  If it has been some time since you engaged in a celebration, get out your calendar and schedule one…and be sure it is a responsibility that appears on your calendar regularly!

## Study Questions

1. What do you believe to be your *purpose?* Do you have ample opportunities to express your purpose?
2. How have hardships in your life contributed to the development and expression of your purpose?
3. What prevents people from recognizing and expressing gratitude to those who have touched their lives?
4. Do you express gratitude freely and often? If not, why not?
5. What do you do for fun? Is it God-honoring?
6. How do you differentiate pleasure, happiness, and joy?
7. How does the popular media offer examples of *joyful* lives?
8. How do you see God bringing joy to your life?

## Related scriptures to pray

Deuteronomy 10:12-13
Psalm 25:15
      37:23-24
      138:8
Proverbs 29:18
Matthew 25:14-29
Romans 8:28
      14:17
2 Thessalonians 1:11

# CHAPTER 9
# PUTTING IT ALL TOGETHER


This book has discussed some of the factors that contribute to holistic health---the integration and wellness of your body, mind, and spirit.  Holistic health is a process, not a fixed entity.  There is no cookie-cutter plan that is right for everyone and there is no miracle substance that you can ingest or program you can complete that will provide you with a state of perfect health (despite what the ads may claim!).  Rather, it is a strategy of *BALANCE* whereby you:

> **B**elieve you can achieve an abundant, empowered life so that you can strengthen positive lifestyle habits and change those patterns that prevent you from achieving optimum health
>
> **A**ssess the current state of your body, mind, and spirit so that you'll understand your unique capabilities and deficits
>
> **L**earn about the meaning of good health and habits that foster it
>
> **A**cquire positive habits that are tailored to your unique body, mind, spirit and lifestyle
>
> **N**urture yourself so that you enhance the ability of your mind and spirit to promote good health
>
> **C**onnect in a better way with yourself, significant others in your life, and Jesus Christ
>
> **E**xperience and learn to appreciate life's blessings so that you can live abundantly

This is a slow and continuous process, but one with profound and long-term benefits.  And the key is that you are seeking balance, not perfection.


After reviewing the various components of a balanced life discussed in this book, you are prepared to consider the degree of balance in your life.  The following pages provide an exercise to guide you through this process.  Begin by plotting where you'd assess yourself to be along the continuum of the 20 items listed on the pages that follow.

## *Assessing Your Balance*

*Plot on each of the following continuums where you assess yourself to be in regard to these various aspects of your life.*

### Relationship with Jesus Christ

| 10 | 5 | 1 |
|---|---|---|
| Accepted Christ as Savior; Strong relationship | Accepted Christ as Savior but occasionally doubt or feel unsure | No relationship with Jesus Christ; unsaved |

### Diet

| 10 | 5 | 1 |
|---|---|---|
| Consistently eat according to food pyramid | <2 Fruits & vegetables daily; eat "junk food" >3 times a week | Rarely eat fruits & vegetables; eat "junk food" daily |

### Fluids

| 10 | 5 | 1 |
|---|---|---|
| Drink 6-8 glasses of water per day; rarely drink soda | Drink 6-8 glasses of water daily; <4 coffees or sodas daily | Drink <3 glasses of water daily; high coffee and/or soda intake |

### Elimination

| 10 | 5 | 1 |
|---|---|---|
| Daily bowel movement without difficulty | Every other day bowel movement without difficulty | Irregularity; dependent on laxatives/enemas |

### Exercise

| 10 | 5 | 1 |
|---|---|---|
| 15 minutes daily or at least 30 minutes 3 times/week | Less than 2 times per week | No regular exercise |

### Sleep/Rest

| 10 | 5 | 1 |
|---|---|---|
| No problem falling or staying asleep; naps <15 minutes | Difficulty falling or staying asleep <3 times/week; irregular naps | Nightly difficulty falling or staying asleep; no naps or frequent naps lasting >30 minutes |

### Sex

| 10 | 5 | 1 |
| --- | --- | --- |
| Level & frequency of intimacy satisfying to self and spouse | Self or spouse dissatisfied with level or frequency | Self or spouse totally disinterested; no intimacy; adulterous; promiscuous |

### Prayer

| 10 | 5 | 1 |
| --- | --- | --- |
| Daily prayer time; weekly church attendance | Irregular prayer; attend church <2 times/month | No prayer life or church attendance |

### Solitude

| 10 | 5 | 1 |
| --- | --- | --- |
| At least 15 minutes of personal time daily; quarterly retreat | At least 15 minutes personal time <3 times/week; yearly retreat | No personal private time |

### Work/Vocation

| 10 | 5 | 1 |
| --- | --- | --- |
| Fully satisfied; using gifts and talents regularly | Occasionally dissatisfied; seldom use gifts and talents | Completely dissatisfied; rarely use gifts and talents |

### Purpose

| 10 | 5 | 1 |
| --- | --- | --- |
| Consistently feel life has meaning and that I have a purpose for living | Regularly question meaning of life and my purpose | Feel hopeless and that I make little difference |

### Leisure

| 10 | 5 | 1 |
| --- | --- | --- |
| Engage in play or hobby daily | Engage in play or hobby weekly | No hobby, seldom play |

### Relationships

| 10 | 5 | 1 |
| --- | --- | --- |
| Satisfying, nurturing, good balance of give and take | Often stressful but more positive than negative | Draining; stressful; negative; abusive |

### Connection with Nature

| 10 | 5 | 1 |
|---|---|---|
| Enjoy nature (trees, birds, etc) >1 hour/week | Enjoy nature <30 minutes weekly | Enjoy nature <1 hour per month |

### Service

| 10 | 5 | 1 |
|---|---|---|
| Consistently have helpful attitude; weekly volunteer activity | Selective helping; occasionally volunteer | Not serving; helping does not come easily |

### Study

| 10 | 5 | 1 |
|---|---|---|
| Read/study Bible daily | Read/study Bible weekly | Rarely read/study Bible |

### Fasting

| 10 | 5 | 1 |
|---|---|---|
| Fast from food or activity at least once/month | Fast from food or activity <3 times/year | No fasting |

### Celebration

| 10 | 5 | 1 |
|---|---|---|
| Joyful life majority of time; regular fellowship and fun | More joyfulness than not; fellowship and fun on major holidays/celebrations | Joyless life; lack fellowship and fun |

### Symptoms

| 10 | 5 | 1 |
|---|---|---|
| Symptom-free | Headaches, pain, indigestion, other symptoms once weekly | Daily symptoms |

### Health Screening

| 10 | 5 | 1 |
|---|---|---|
| Prompt attention to symptoms; physical/dental/eye exams within past year<br>*Female:* annual mammogram, monthly self-exam of breasts<br>*Male:* monthly self-exam of testicles | Delay having symptoms evaluated; exams 1-3 years; self-exams every 2-3 month | Ignore symptoms; >3 years since last exams; no self-exams |

Place dots on your score for each item on this Balance Wheel:

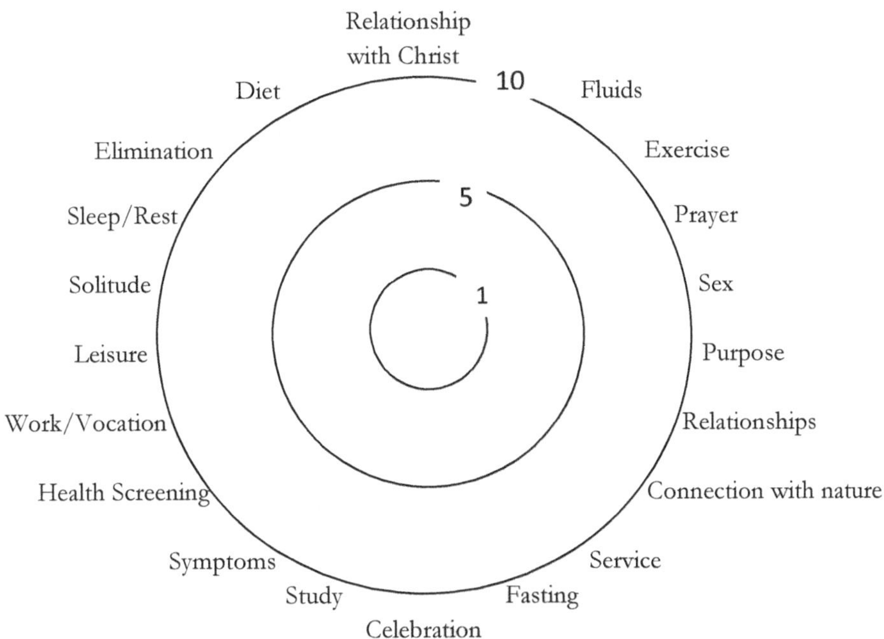


Now connect the dots.

You may find that your Balance Wheel lacks a completely smooth surface. Some of these imbalances may merely create minor bumps in your journey that are hardly noticeable, although in time, they can risk throwing your total being out of alignment. Others may be sufficiently deep that they are obviously disrupting your health and well-being now. Your challenge is to take responsibility for restoring and maintaining balance so that you can enjoy optimal holistic health. This begins by taking stock of where your major imbalances exist. Look over your Balance Wheel and list areas of imbalance:

Now, prioritize them. In your prioritization, consider imbalances that are causing the most interference with your ability to achieve optimal health and your fullest relationship with the Lord. Write the three areas that lead your list of imbalances:

1.

2.

3.

Look at the imbalances you identified, think about them, and pray about them. Tell God that you want to change these aspects of your life and ask Him for guidance on the best means to do so. Spend some time meditating to hear what He may offer.

Develop a plan for improving these three imbalances. Consider the goals or outcomes you want to achieve, actions that can assist you in getting there, and reasonable dates for achieving them. You can review chapters in this book that discuss specific areas to obtain some suggestions. Write your plan in a format similar to this:

| Imbalance | Goal | Actions | Target Date |
|---|---|---|---|
|  |  |  |  |
|  |  |  |  |
|  |  |  |  |

Pray that God will help you to achieve these goals and reveal to you any changes that you need to make in your plans.

Develop a list of affirmations related to your goals. For example, if one of your goals is to spend 30 minutes walking in the park twice each week, state this in the form of an affirmative statement that puts you in the place of actually achieving it: *I spend 30 minutes walking in the park two times each week.* This sets a standard for you to achieve and conveys to your brain a message that you are actively engaging in the act. Write down these affirmations and place a copy where you will regularly see it, so that they will be active in your thoughts. Continue praying for God's assistance.

Your intention and actions to address your imbalances should help you to improve these areas of your life. You can then revisit your Balance Wheel and address other priorities.

There certainly are many health benefits to achieving holistic health through balance, such as feeling and functioning at your best and preventing illness. But, there also are other, very powerful advantages that Christians need to consider in promoting optimal holistic health:

- To honor God and the temple He has given you
- To live an abundant life that enables you to serve Him
- To serve as a model to the world of a life enriched by a relationship with Jesus Christ

May you be empowered by the Lord to realize your best and enjoy the fruits of holistic health.

# NOTES

1. Foster RJ and Griffin E. Spiritual Classics. Selected Readings for Individuals and Groups on the  Twelve Spiritual Disciplines. New York: HarperSanFrancisco, 2007.

2. Uchino BN, Cacioppo JR, and Kiecolt-Glaser JK. The relationship between social support and physiological processes.  A review with emphasis on underlying mechanisms and implications for health. Psychological bulletin, 119: 488-531, 1996.

3. George LK. Social factors and the onset and outcome of depression.  In KW Schaie, D Blazer, and JS House (eds), Aging, Health Behaviors, and Health Outcomes, pp 137-159).  Hillsdale, NJ: Lawrence Erlbaum Associates, 1992.

4. Berkman L. The role of social relations in health promotion.  Psychosomatic Medicine 57:245-254, 1995.

5. Spiegel D. et al.  Effect of psychosocial treatment on survival of patients with metastatic breast cancer. Lancer 2: 888-891, 1989.

6. Sapolsky RM, Alberts SC, and Altman J.  Hypercortisolism associated with social subordinance or social isolation among wild baboons.  Archives of General Psychiatry, 54: 1137-1143, 1997.

7. Foster, R.  Celebration of Discipline, 3rd ed., San Francisco: Harper Collins, 2002.

8. Willard, D.  The Divine Conspiracy:  Rediscovering Our Hidden Life in God,  San Francisco: HarperSanFrancisco,  p418, 1998.

9. Payne, L.  Listening Prayer.  Learning to Hear God's Voice and Keep a Prayer Journal,  Grand Rapids, MI: Baker Books, 2000, p58-59.

10. Marshall, C.  A Closer Walk.  *Old* Tappan, NJ:  Chosen Books/Revell, 1986.

11. Willard, D.  The Spirit of the Disciplines.  Understanding How God Changes Lives, , San    Francisco: HarperSanFrancisco, p. 167, 1990.

ABOUT THE AUTHOR:
# Charlotte Eliopoulos RN, MPH, ND, PhD

A respected and prolific author, Charlotte has written over a dozen books and numerous chapters and articles related to geriatrics and holistic health.  Through her writings and workshops, she has equipped individuals to achieve maximum physical, mental, and spiritual health and well-being.

Charlotte holds degrees in nursing, naturopathy, and public health.  She can be reached at charlotte@healthed.net.